The Winnowing of White Witchcraft

I0893974

MEDIEVAL AND RENAISSANCE TEXTS AND STUDIES

VOLUME 512

MRTS TEXTS FOR TEACHING

VOLUME 10

The Winnowing of White Witchcraft

Edward Poeton

Edited with an introduction and notes
by
Simon F. Davies

ARIZONA CENTER FOR MEDIEVAL
ACMRS
AND RENAISSANCE STUDIES

Tempe, Arizona
2018

THE ARIZONA CENTER FOR
MEDIEVAL & RENAISSANCE
STUDIES

Published by ACMRS (Arizona Center for Medieval and Renaissance Studies)
Tempe, Arizona
© 2018 Arizona Board of Regents for Arizona State University.
All Rights Reserved.

Library of Congress Cataloging-in-Publication Data

Names: Poeton, Edward, author. | Davies, Simon F., editor.
Title: The winnowing of white witchcraft / Edward Poeton ; edited with an introduction and notes by Simon F. Davies.
Description: Tempe : Arizona Center for Medieval and Renaissance Studies, 2018. | Series: Medieval and Renaissance texts and studies ; Volume 512 | Includes bibliographical references and index.
Identifiers: LCCN 2017029557 | ISBN 9780866985673 (paperback : alk. paper)
Subjects: LCSH: Witchcraft--History--16th century. | Witchcraft--History--17th century.
Classification: LCC BF1571 .P63 2017 | DDC 133.4/3--dc23
LC record available at https://lccn.loc.gov/2017029557

Cover Art:
Book of magic, with instructions for invoking spirits, etc. (ca. 1577–1583)
Folger Shakespeare Library V.b.26 (1).
Licensed under CC BY-SA 4.0
https://creativecommons.org/licenses/by-sa/4.0

∞

This book is made to last. It is set in Adobe Caslon Pro,
and printed on acid-free paper to library specifications.
Printed in the United States of America

Contents

Acknowledgments

My biggest debt of gratitude incurred in the production of this edition is to Jenny Richards, who introduced me to Poeton and his *Winnowing* in the first place, the day before I submitted my doctoral thesis. Jenny has been consistently supportive of my career and I am in her debt. Many thanks are due to the British Library, who hold the manuscript, and to whom I am grateful for permission to reproduce this edited transcript and the two images of it. Further thanks, for invaluable assistance provided along the way, go to Paul Quinn, Christopher Whittick, Jennifer Evans, Richard Coates, and Margaret Healy. I am also very grateful to Ross Dandridge, whose work in this area has saved me a great deal of labor, and to whom I wish the very best in his future research. Finally, I wish to thank Medieval and Renaissance Texts and Studies for taking the edition on, Roy Rukkila for his careful copy-editing, and the two anonymous reviewers for their kind and thoughtful comments.

Introduction

Poeton's Life and Writings

Very little is known about the life of Edward Poeton. With one minor exception his writings on a variety of subjects were never published in print, including his treatise on witchcraft, of which this is the first print edition. Perhaps as a result Poeton has received very little attention in the voluminous historiography of English witchcraft belief; although Keith Thomas (in this, as in so many things, a pioneer) mentioned *The Winnowing of White Witchcraft* as an "excellent account of the activities of a seventeenth-century wizard, seen through the eyes of a contemporary medical practitioner."[1] The most extensive analysis of Poeton's work is in a recent doctoral thesis by Ross Dandridge, which examines Poeton in the context of early seventeenth-century anti-quack literature.[2] It is the hope of the editor that this edition will go some way towards rectifying this neglect, given the work's particular interest as the only treatise of its kind dedicated solely to attacking the "good" witch, or white witch.

Poeton describes himself as "Licentiate in Physick and Chyrurgery," meaning that though he was primarily a physician (and that he had a license to practice) he also practiced surgery, as many physicians did.[3] We know that Poeton lived and practiced medicine in London, for a time at least, until shortly before the death of his master Thomas Bonham, when he moved to Petworth in West Sussex. Hints in the *Winnowing* suggest that Poeton may also have lived in Suffolk at some time. Poeton is a rare name in England, though it can be traced back to the fourteenth century, where it appears in the West Country; if there is a connection this may suggest an originating locale for the name.[4] Edward does not appear to have attended university, although there is a slim chance he may

---

1 Keith Thomas, *Religion and the Decline of Magic* (London: Weidenfeld & Nicolson, 1971), 252, bibliographical note.

2 Ross Dandridge, "Anti-Quack Literature in Early Stuart England" (unpublished Ph.D. thesis, Queen Mary, University of London, 2012). Available online at https://qmro.qmul.ac.uk.

3 Thomas Bonham, *The Chyrvrgians Closet* (London: George Miller for Edward Brester, 1630), a3^{r}; see also the title page of *The Midwives Deputie*, §1 in British Library Sloane MS 1954.

4 National Archives C 241/43/99.

be the Edward Payton of Warwick who matriculated at Hart Hall, Oxford, in November 1594, aged 18; Payton is a potential variant spelling of Poeton.[5] This cannot, however, be confirmed, and if Poeton had had a degree it seems likely that he would have mentioned it, given how proudly he announces his status as "Licentiate" (and how keen he is to establish, in one of the anecdotes he recounts, that its protagonist is Master of Arts, as well as like the author "*Licenciate* bothe in *Physick and chyrurgerie*," 24). Poeton was married and had at least one child, John, who matriculated at St. Alban Hall, Oxford, in 1637, aged 18, and who went on to a career in the church. John died in 1692 in Withyham, Sussex, where he was minister.[6] Edward Poeton died in 1644, and was buried in Petworth parish church.

Petworth, where Poeton ended his days, and where he wrote the *Winnowing*, is a small town with a population at the time of around a thousand.[7] Poeton seems to have been practicing as a physician there by 1626; he may have had an existing connection there with Sir Henry Dawtry, a member of the local gentry, to whom the *Winnowing* is dedicated.[8] We know that there was interest in witchcraft at the local manor, Petworth House, where the library of Henry Percy, the ninth earl of Northumberland, was well-stocked with Continental treatises on the subject, some of them annotated by the earl. Indeed, the ninth earl came to be known as the "wizard" earl, although his interest in the occult has been overstated.[9] There is no evidence that the earl took any interest in this lowly physician who moved to Petworth shortly before Percy's death in 1632, and Poeton's work shows no influence of the Continental demonology the earl clearly took an interest in. Petworth is a very small town, however, and the manor house is located in the center of it; it is intriguing to consider the proximity of two men so interested in this subject. Poeton's *The Midwives Deputie*, also in Sloane MS 1954, is dedicated to Anne, Countess of Northumberland, wife of the tenth earl, so at the very least we know that Poeton sought patronage from the family, whether or not he

[5] Another possible variant spelling is Poulton, and there is an Edward Poulton who also graduated from Hart Hall in 1568; he would be just about the right age, but any concrete identification with either seems unlikely. Joseph Foster, *Alumni Oxonienses: The Members of the University of Oxford, 1500–1714*, 4 vols. (London: James Parker, 1891), III, 1131, 1189.

[6] Foster, *Alumni Oxonienses*, III, 1175; National Archives PROB 11/409/101.

[7] On Petworth, see G. H. Kenyon, "Petworth Town & Trades 1610–1760," *Sussex Archaeological Collections*, 96 (1958): 35–107; Andy Wood, "'Some banglyng about the customes': Popular Memory and the Experience of Defeat in a Sussex Village, 1549–1640," *Rural History*, 25, 1 (2014): 1–14. For the county-wide medical context, see D. A. Beaufort, "The Medical Practitioners of Western Sussex in the Early Modern Period: A Preliminary Survey," *Sussex Archaeological Collections*, 131 (1993): 139–51.

[8] Dandridge, "Anti-Quack Literature," 120.

[9] G. R. Batho, "The Library of the 'Wizard' Earl: Henry Percy Ninth Earl of Northumberland (1564–1632)," *The Library*, 15, 4 (1960): 246–61.

obtained it. The dedication appears to indicate that Poeton's only actual contact with the countess was his having seen her in church.

Poeton's only known appearance in print was as editor of his former master Thomas Bonham's medical papers, published as *The Chyrvrgians Closet* (1630), to which Poeton provided two brief dedications and an even briefer note to the reader. As Poeton explains in the latter:

> I was a long (and the last) seruant, vnto the Right Worshipfull, M^r^. THOMAS BONHAM D^r^. of Physick . . . who whilest he liued was to me a Master, yea more, a Father, and at his death a bountifull Benefactor; for he gaue and deliuered vnto mee before he dyed, all his Manuscripts, both of Physicke and Chyrurgerie[.][10]

Bonham, who died in 1628, was involved in a protracted dispute with the Royal College of Physicians in the early part of the century, because he practiced medicine without a license from the College (having been refused admittance) and repeatedly refused to desist from doing so. Bonham persistently took the side of the Barber-Surgeons' Company against the College of Physicians, with whom they were in competition.[11] One of the dedications Poeton added to the edition of Bonham's papers was to the Barber-Surgeons, so it is clear that he was following his late master in this respect.

Poeton did, however, leave behind four treatises in manuscript, as well as what has been termed a commonplace book, all now in the Sloane collection in the British Library.[12] The commonplace book, Sloane MS 1965, is a lengthy compendium of a variety of material (around 180 leaves in folio), though not all of it is in Poeton's hand. Poeton's name is on the first leaf, and the (modern) Sloane collection binding gives it the title "E. Poeton. Medical Collections." The collection includes astrological information (some of which is signed by a Phillip Prowse), a large medical treatise titled "Of the necessitie profitt and prais of phisicke" (largely a compendium of remedies and recipes), a treatise on the four humours, "material gathered out of [Robert Burton's] the Anatomy of Melancholy," a collection of epigrams, songs and other quotations, medical receipts, herbal notes, and medical recipes. Only the medical treatise and the treatise on the humours seem to be in Poeton's hand (if it is indeed his hand; see below), so they should more accurately be described as further additions to his works. The

---

10 Bonham, *The Chyrvrgians Closet*, a4^r^.

11 See George Clark, *A History of the Royal College of Physicians of London*, 3 vols. (Oxford: Clarendon Press, 1964), I, 208–10; Harold J. Cook, "Bonham, Thomas (*c.* 1564–*c.* 1628)" in *ODNB*.

12 On Sir Hans Sloane and his collections, see Arthur MacGregor, ed., *Sir Hans Sloane: Collector, Scientist, Antiquary* (London: British Museum Press, 1994).

collection as a whole was presumably put together at a later date. The subtitle of the medical treatise explains that:

> this booke containeth most notable rare p[ro]fitable & pretious medicines for al accidentse and infirmities y^{t} are incidente unto all inwarde & outwarde p[ar]ts of mans body ye approued secrets of many learned men who haue imparted ye same unto me & some wch I haue found out by mine owne studie and experienced practice[.][13]

It includes remedies for a huge range of conditions, including madness, dropsy, shingles, the stitch, and hangovers.[14]

Poeton's most original and most important work, however, is to be found in the four treatises now bound together as Sloane MS 1954. The collection is in the uniform Sloane library binding and is given the fairly accurate title "Medical Treatises." All four are in folio and are fair copies written out in a neat secretary hand (see Figure 1). It is possible that the manuscripts are the work of a professional scribe, but given the nature of many of the corrections made to the treatises (which seem clearly to be the work of their author) and the correspondence with the less formally-presented treatises in the "commonplace book" it seems, on balance, most likely that the hand of Sloane MS 1954 is Poeton's own.

The first and longest tract in the collection is *The Midwives Deputie. Or A holp for such as are not well furnished wth knowledg concerning the misteries of ye profession*. The subtitle adds that the work is "*published for a further help, vnto such as are desirous to take paynes in ye profession*." As the dedication makes clear, Poeton wrote the treatise for his wife, who was "a sworne midwife."[15] It is compiled, he writes, both from the work of other authors and from his own experience, though the former seems to make up the bulk of it. The treatise is a dialogue between a midwife and her deputy. It discusses the nature and history of the midwife's craft, as well as offering extensive guidance on its practice, via directions for preparation for the birth itself, remedies for problems that might arise, and methods of diagnosing those problems. The work foreshadows the concerns of the *Winnowing* in a number of interesting ways, most significantly in Poeton's concern throughout that the midwife should be educated: "a woman well read, and well experienced in this matter." The midwife character regularly supports her arguments with scriptural quotations, demonstrating a degree of education, and is keen to show her license and explain the articles that it contains, which a midwife was sworn to observe.[16] It is clear that this treatise is fully in accord with Poeton's arguments against uneducated medical practitioners in the *Winnowing*. He also attempted

---

13 British Library Sloane MS 1965, fol. 20^{r}.

14 Sloane MS 1965, fols. 24^{r}, 53^{r}, 36^{r}, 46^{v}, 24^{v}.

15 Sloane MS 1954, §1, ¶2^{r}.

16 Sloane MS 1954, §1, ¶3^{r}, 6.

to make the work accessible, explaining that "in the manner I haue striuen wth my self to vse the most ordinary words and the playnest phrases, to express the matter by that I coulde deuise." In both form and intention Poeton exhibits his desire to share his knowledge and experience with others, a desire which lies behind all of his output, and the forms that he chooses. "And thus much I profess," he states, "that I wish the knowledg of all such things (as may safely be vsed) that will doe good, that they were even as common as the light."[17]

The second treatise in the volume is *The ordering of yong children*, which is intended as an addition to the first. It is mentioned on the title page of *The Midwives Deputie*, and does not have a separate title page of its own. It is also a dialogue, with the same characters as the preceding treatise, and follows directly on from it. *The ordering of yong children* deals with such issues as choosing a nurse for the child, how to clean the child and, for the majority of the work, how to deal with the various ailments and illnesses to which newborn babies are susceptible.

The third tract in the collection is a polemic against uroscopy, or uromancy, which is the process of diagnosing illness from a visual examination of the patient's urine. This treatise is entitled *The Vrinall crackt in the carriage. Or a tract asserting the impossibilitie of diseases right discerning: by a carryed vrines bare inspection*—a urinal referring to a container in which urine was transported. This tract has the most relevance to the current edition, as we shall see, for it touches on many of the same areas. During the medieval period, uroscopy had been a commonly-used and trusted weapon in the physician's arsenal, but by the seventeenth century the practice was largely discredited, at least among educated physicians. It was still widely practiced, however, both by some unscrupulous physicians and by a wide range of unlicensed medical practitioners.[18] While Poeton, in accord with his educated colleagues, allows that examination of a patient's urine can indicate certain things about the liver, the kidneys, the bladder, and the blood, he allows it no further efficacy than this. In particular he is very keen to stress that examination of urine must be carried out immediately after it is passed and in the house in which the patient is located, rather than being transported. The unreliability of transporting urine—the "absurd custom of pissportage," as he calls it—is among Poeton's main objections to the practice, as indicated by the title of the tract.[19] Even the diagnosis of problems with the aforementioned body parts—parts of the body to which urine is related—is highly uncertain on the examination of urine alone; therefore, it is utterly ridiculous, Poeton argues, to diagnose problems with the brain, heart, lungs, etc., from urine, and even more

---

17 Sloane MS 1954, §1, ¶3[r], 31.

18 See Lucinda McCray Beier, *Sufferers and Healers: The Experience of Illness in Seventeenth-Century England* (London: Routledge and Kegan Paul, 1987), 40–41; Michael Stolberg, "The Decline of Uroscopy in Early Modern Learned Medicine (1500–1650)," *Early Science and Medicine*, 12, 3 (2007): 313–36.

19 Sloane MS 1954, §3, 1, 2.

so if that urine has been carried far from the patient in a dirty vessel. True medical diagnosis, Poeton argues (fairly reasonably), is a lot more complex than this.[20] Uroscopy, however, seems to have been a popular service. Poeton writes:

> our country Corydons, (wth one vne-animall consent) haue caught it vp for a custome, to carry their waters vp and downe the country, to this or that cunning man, cunning woman, Quack, knaue, or else to some potent Parson Pissprophet, from whom they expect no less then a Delphian oracle. Clottishly conceiuing, that any Artist is able, from out the bare inspection of a ported pispot, to discerne, discouer, and dicipher, the sick mans state, wth all the seuerall symptomes, of each sicknes whatsoeuer.[21]

Poeton was by no means the only physician to attack the subject during this period, and a number of other tracts, to which Poeton refers, had already been published.[22] They formed part of the wider attack on unlicensed and unlearned medical practitioners, discussed further below. The figures mentioned in the above quotation were key targets of this wider campaign; they also recur as targets of Poeton's wrath in the final tract in the collection, *The Winnowing of White Witchcraft*.

The exact dating of the treatises, and their order of composition, is not clear. The *Winnowing* definitely post-dates 1631, as it refers to two works on the weapon-salve published in that year. Poeton's engagement with the weapon-salve controversy (see below) might lead one to assume that the work was published shortly after this date, while the debate was still a topical issue; he clearly feels the need to make his thoughts on the subject plain, even though it is a slight departure from the main issues of the work. We know, however, that *The Midwives Deputie* and *The Vrinall* were written later than this, the former definitely in 1637, as both refer to works published that year; *The Midwives Deputie* is dedicated to Anne, Countess of Northumberland, who died that year, so cannot be any later. Dandridge suggests that the remaining treatises followed closely in the wake of *The Midwives Deputie*.[23] However, the binding of Sloane MS 1954 is not contemporary, therefore there is no reason to assume that the current ordering of the tracts is the original one. *The Midwives Deputie* and *The Vrinall* use paper with the same watermark, while *The ordering of yong Children* and *The Winnowing* share paper with a different watermark, perhaps indicating that they were written at a different time—though the former at least was presumably written later

20 Sloane MS 1954, §3, 28, 21–33.

21 Sloane MS 1954, §3, 2.

22 Pieter van Foreest, *The Arraignment Of Vrines*, trans. James Hart (London: George Eld for Robert Milbourne, 1623); James Hart, *The Anatomie Of Vrines* (London: Richard Field for Robert Milbourne, 1625); Thomas Brian, *The Pisse-Prophet, Or, Certaine Pisse-Pot Lectures* (London: E. P. for R. Thrale, 1637).

23 Dandridge, "Anti-Quack Literature," 121–22.

than *The Midwives Deputie*, as it is a sequel to it. The presentation of the treatises is generally uniform, though with marked differences in ink between the treatises. The evidence of whether or not *The Vrinall* precedes the *Winnowing* is in fact inconclusive, although it seems more probable that it does: Poeton refers to "another tract called the unmasking of urines uncertaynties" in his preface to the *Winnowing* (6), which would seem to confirm that this tract is the later one. However, this is not the *Vrinall*'s title, so he was perhaps still working on at least that part of it while writing the *Winnowing*. He also has his characters refer to "our last conference . . . about urines uncertaynties" (9), again using the wrong title, and implying that the other treatise is a dialogue similar to the *Winnowing*, which it is not. Poeton had certainly not said all he had to say on the subject of uromancy, as he returns to the issue repeatedly throughout the *Winnowing*. Overall, however, a date sometime in the 1630s, probably towards the end of the decade, seems to be as precise as we are likely to get in this respect, and it seems most likely, though not certain, that the *Winnowing* was the latest of the tracts to be completed.

The Winnowing of White Witchcraft

Of all the four treatises in Sloane MS 1954, *The Winnowing of White Witchcraft* has the most elaborate title page (see figure 2). It is also the most fully-developed in terms of structure: while the first two tracts are also dialogues, they do not have named characters as the *Winnowing* does nor are the characters so fully realized. Like the others, the treatise is a fair copy (i.e., not a first or rough draft), and seems intended for publication—if not for print then at least for circulating to others in its current form. The title page certainly suggests as much. The treatise includes catchwords on each page, perhaps suggesting that it was the author's intention to have it bound by a professional binder. Why it was never printed is not known—there is no evidence that Poeton had any interest in printing his work, so it may never have been intended to be printed—but it is at least worthy of note that it is not the only witchcraft treatise from around this time to survive in manuscript that was not printed during the period: Edward Fairfax's *Daemonologia* (1621) also did not see print, and in this instance it seems the author may well have wished that it had.[24] There are also no known news pamphlets reporting cases of witchcraft from these decades, and it has been suggested by some scholars that interest in the subject was fading during these years (to be re-ignited in the 1640s in the wake of Matthew Hopkins' witch hunt in East

[24] Edward Fairfax, *Daemonologia: A Discourse on Witchcraft*, ed. William Grainge (London: Frederick Muller, 1971).

Anglia) and perhaps, if Poeton ever did consider printing the work, there was simply not the market for it.[25]

As well as Poeton's own relatively sparse marginal headings, the *Winnowing* is annotated throughout in the margin by a second hand, the only one of the four treatises to be so annotated. These notes have not been reproduced in this edition, as they are not by Poeton; rather than being part of the treatise itself they should more accurately be considered consanguineous with the sort of annotations made by readers in early modern printed books. They are indeed typical of such annotations—in general either drawing attention to useful *sententiae* or soundbites, or providing headings which merely summarize the text in order to aid navigation through the work. Occasionally they offer a value judgement. Sometimes they expand on Poeton's own marginal notes: for example, on page 24, where Poeton's note simply reads "A History," the secondary annotator adds: "of a white wich of stoke clare a pryory house in Suffolk." Several such expansions are made throughout. The secondary annotator sometimes gets things wrong, thus proving that the notes are not by Poeton. For example, they gloss a reference to King Saul's visit to "a woman who had a familiar spirit" with the note: "King Saul had a Familliar spirit"; this annotator's knowledge of the subject was clearly not extensive, and the notes were surely made after the treatise had left Poeton's hands. Overall, the most interesting thing about these notes is their existence: they indicate that it was read fairly closely by another, who had the intention of either returning to the text themselves or of circulating it to others. And given that similar annotations do not appear in the other treatises in the volume, they perhaps indicate that this subject was of more interest to others than the other subjects on which Poeton wrote.

The Winnowing of White Witchcraft is a dialogue between three characters: a divine, a physician, and a country bumpkin (see Figure 1). The latter represents the "student" character of the dialogue, an uneducated person who is sinning without realizing it and is reformed over the course of the conversation. The other two characters are Poeton's mouthpieces, offering, in accord with their professions, theological and medical arguments. The dialogue form was popular among writers on witchcraft: George Gifford, Henry Holland, and James I had all used it in their treatises on the subject; Gifford and James claimed they did so in order to make their treatises more accessible, and this seems likely to have been Poeton's rationale too.[26] The form also had a long tradition in Continental

[25] James Sharpe calls witchcraft "a dying subject" in the 1630s, *Instruments of Darkness—Witchcraft in England 1550–1750* (London: Penguin, 1997), 146. For a good overview of such issues, see also Malcolm Gaskill, "Witchcraft and Evidence in Early Modern England," *Past and Present*, 198 (2008): 33–70.

[26] George Gifford, *A Dialogve concerning Witches and Witchcraftes* (London: John Windet for Toby Cooke and Mihil Hart, 1593), A3r; James VI and I, *Daemonologie* (Edinburgh: Robert Waldegrave, 1597), A2v.

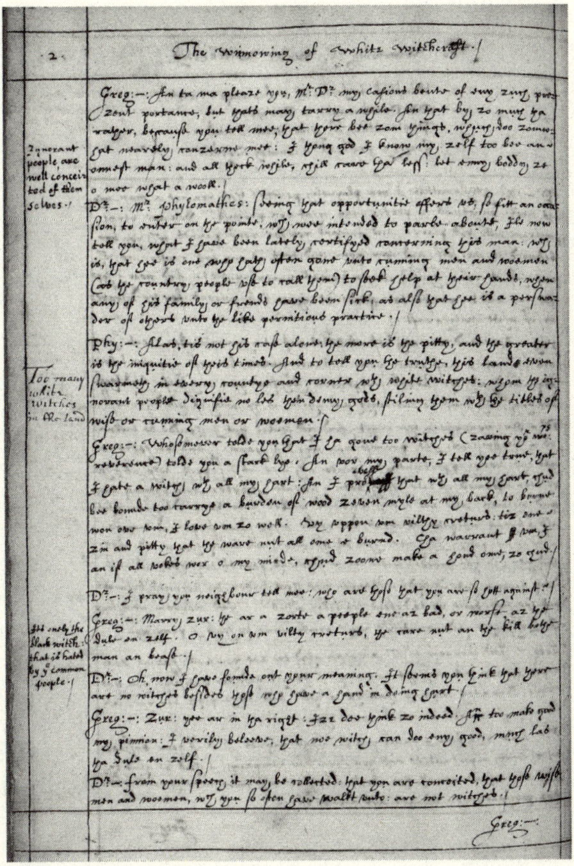

Fig 1: Page from *The Winnowing of White Wichcraft* © The British Library Board (Sloane MS 1954, fol. 164v).

demonology. It was by no means limited to writing on witchcraft, however, and was popular among English reformers much more widely, particularly because of its capacity to appeal to less-educated audiences. George Gifford, for example, used the form for several of his most popular works.[27] Gifford's use of the dialogue form in his *Dialogve concerning Witches and Witchcraftes* (1593) is the most developed example of the form in writing on witchcraft, although Poeton's comes a close second, and is the most similar to Poeton's found in print. Gifford may well have been an influence on Poeton, although there is no conclusive evidence that the latter had read the earlier work. Like Poeton's, Gifford's dialogue features more than the customary two characters (usually just master and student),

[27] See A. B. Zlatar, *Reformation Fictions: Polemical Protestant Dialogues in Elizabethan England* (Oxford: Oxford University Press, 2011).

one of whom is a rustic and a regular client of cunning folk, just like Poeton's Gregory Groshead. (Gifford also includes this character's wife and her friend in order to represent extremes of stubbornness.) Poeton's dialogue is unusual in having two educated characters to represent the twin poles of divinity and medicine. The separation is an important one, as we shall see. The divine's arguments predominantly revolve around extensive citation of scripture in support of his exhortations against visiting cunning folk. He is a less successful debater than the divine in Gifford's *Dialogve*, who demonstrates a better understanding of potential counter-arguments. Presumably this results from the fact that Poeton was not himself a divine; he is on strongest ground when arguing for the benefits of education in matters of healing and when discussing his experiences as a physician.

Gregory Groshead describes himself as a "playne cuntry man" and at one point requests that the divine use simpler language (28). As with the yokel characters in Gifford's dialogue, Gregory, although an exaggerated stereotype of a countryman, may be intended to offer answers which prepare Poeton's readers—from among the clergy and his fellow physicians, for example—for the kinds of responses they can expect to receive from their parishioners and clients. That is, the treatise may be aimed as much at Poeton's peers as it is intended to be didactic to ordinary folk like Gregory. As well as making the treatise easier to read in its own right, Gregory's request for the Doctor to simplify his discourse may be a reminder to these readers to fit their language to their audience. It is also, no doubt, intended to be entertaining, and Gregory is certainly intended to be a source of humor to Poeton's readers. Although Gregory grows tetchy at some points, in general he is an extremely patient student and eventually is convinced of the error of his ways.

A particularly notable feature of the presentation of Gregory is that he speaks in an exaggerated regional dialect. This was not new in English literature—a famous contemporary example of dialect writing appears in *King Lear*, and the practice goes back to Chaucer's *Reeve's Tale*—but its use in a scholarly treatise is highly unusual. To give an example:

> But vor my parte, (an grace a God) vrom hence vorward, chill bee shure too ze my prayers every morning whanz dee rize: I: an sarve God all tha de after. An than I hope God wooll bless mee vrom tha d'vle. An won thing moore chill veth vully promis ee: that chill nere goe no moore to enny o theise wise vokes agen: zo I woante, nut I.

This would be roughly "translated" into modern English as follows:

> But for my part, (and [with the] grace of God) from hence forward, I'll be sure to say my prayers every morning when us do rise: aye, and serve God all the day after. And then I hope God will bless me from the devil. And

> one thing more I'll faithfully promise you: that I'll never go no more to any of these wise folks again: so I won't, not I.

The dialect may prove difficult to some modern readers, especially those not familiar with English regional accents; the simplest way to deal with it is to read it out loud, as the spellings are largely phonetic (though certain pre-vowel shift vowel sounds such as "ze" and "de" for "say" and "day" should be borne in mind). It has only been very lightly modernized in this edition, given the literary and linguistic interest these passages have. A particularly unfamiliar feature may be the use of "ich," an obsolete form of "I," abbreviated to "ch" and elided with a following word (so "I will" is written "chill"); this is a hangover from Middle English still in use in certain regional dialects during the early modern period. If the dialect is intended to have a specific regional origin, it is unclear; it bears most resemblance to a stereotypical West Country accent—and Poeton may possibly have had roots in the West Country, as already mentioned.[28] There may be some Sussex influence, but only light, if at all. Overall it is not specific enough to be securely identified, and in any case it is exaggerated and may never have been intended to be particularly realistic. Gregory is a generic "yokel" character, and there is no sense of documentary truth to his accent.

Gregory's speeches also include nonce-words (such as "argation" for "argument," 21) and malapropisms (such as "destructions" for "instructions" and "desolved" for "resolved," 22, 73). On several occasions he gets the physician's name wrong—Phylomathes (a commonly-used name in scholarly dialogues) becomes "Phymolathes," an indication at the level of the narrative that Gregory is too simple to pronounce a lengthy Latinate word (even though it is his friend's name), and on the figurative level it tells us something about his character: Gregory is no philomath. The purpose of the dialect passages seems primarily to make the treatise entertaining to its readers; there is certainly a rather unpleasant element of laughter at the expense of the ignorant bumpkin. Whatever the reason, Poeton takes them quite seriously: on a number of occasions he corrects himself when he forgets to write in dialect. Although primarily a literary device intended to be humorous, the dialect passages may also have a serious point. If difficult to understand at times, for example, perhaps this is to make the point that city-educated physicians and clerics may indeed find it difficult to argue with people such as Gregory, but this should be no barrier to doing so. Just as in Gifford's *Dialogve*, which ends with "The good wife R." entering and making a mockery of all that has gone before, readers are alerted to the fact that there will always be others

[28] Stanley Wells suggests that Edgar's dialect passages in *King Lear*, which bear a certain similarity to Gregory's, are intended to represent a West Country accent; see Stanley Wells, ed. *The Oxford Shakespeare: King Lear* (Oxford: Oxford University Press, 2000), 20.227–34 and notes (4.5.234–41 in the folio text).

who remain unconvinced.[29] Although intended to be humorous, the scene that closes Gifford's treatise surely makes a serious point about the difficulties facing those who would "reform" the "common sort," and there may be something similar at work in Poeton's *Winnowing*.

Context: Witchcraft, Medicine, and Magic

To turn now to the themes of the treatise, it is necessary to place it in its context in three main areas: witchcraft, medicine, and ritual magic.

In Europe during the sixteenth and seventeenth centuries thousands of people were tried and often executed for the crime of practicing witchcraft. The traditional definition of witchcraft is the power to cause harm through supernatural means, known in medieval and early modern Europe as *maleficium*. Scholars of late medieval and early modern Europe located the source of this power in a contract with the Devil, this being the worst aspect of the crime in their view. The vast majority of people, however, right across Europe, were concerned—when they were concerned about witchcraft at all—about the harm caused rather than the source of the power. Accusations of witchcraft overwhelmingly revolved around specific misfortunes alleged to have been caused by the accused.[30] England was in fact a region with little interest in witchcraft; current estimates suggest no more than 500 executions in the entire period, and the majority of trials ended in the acquittal of the accused.[31] Treatises on the subject did not sell well. Before Poeton wrote, the largest single trial took place in Lancashire in 1612, in which twelve people were executed, but this was unusual. Accusations tended to revolve around petty local disputes, often in relation to competition for scarce resources. Those accused of witchcraft usually seem to have had bad reputations stretching back many years—recourse to law was a last resort, relying on a particular concatenation of misfortunes and circumstances.

---

[29] Gifford, *Dialogve*, M3^{r}–M4^{v}.

[30] The historiography of witchcraft is very large. Good places to begin are: Simon F. Davies, "Superstition and Witchcraft," in Matthew Dimmock, Andrew Hadfield, and Abigail Shinn, eds., *The Ashgate Research Companion to Popular Culture in Early Modern England* (Farnham: Ashgate, 2014); Sharpe, *Instruments of Darkness*; Brian P. Levack, ed., *The Oxford Handbook of Witchcraft in Early Modern Europe and Colonial America* (Oxford: Oxford University Press, 2013); Robin Briggs, *Witches & Neighbours—The Social and Cultural Context of European Witchcraft* (2nd ed.; Oxford: Blackwell, 2002); Brian P. Levack, *The Witch-Hunt in Early Modern Europe* (3rd ed.; Harlow: Pearson Education Ltd., 2006).

[31] James Sharpe, "England," in Richard M. Golden, ed., *Encyclopedia of Witchcraft—The Western Tradition*, 4 vols. (Santa Barbara: ABC-CLIO, 2006), 411; Sharpe, *Instruments*, chap. 4.

In England, uniquely, witches were said to have spirit companions known as familiars, which usually took the form of animals. In scholarly discourse these were said to be evil spirits or devils, and it was usually through the intercession of a familiar spirit that the diabolic compact was said to have been arranged and sealed. Familiars supposedly drank blood from their owners, and the teat from which they drank, or the mark they left having done so, became known as the witches' or Devil's mark, left to seal the diabolical compact. Familiars took the form of an enormously wide range of animals; they also occasionally appeared in human form.[32]

As well as harmful witches, there were also figures known as white witches—otherwise known as cunning folk, wise men/women, good witches, etc.—and it is with such figures that Poeton is concerned in this treatise, as its title indicates. While the evidence is uncertain as to whether or not any of those accused of being harmful witches actually believed in their own powers, white witches really existed and offered a commercial service which many early modern people found very useful. Their services included finding lost or stolen goods, healing both humans and animals, love potions, and diagnosing and curing bewitchment from black witches (as well as identifying the witch—evidence which was sometimes used in trials). White witches were predominantly male and were concentrated in towns and cities, though they were found throughout the country.[33] Poeton also includes astrologers in his definition of white witches; although in many ways separate spheres of activity, practitioners of beneficial magic often offered astrological services as well. There are several well-known contemporary examples of the sort of figure Poeton has in mind, such as Simon Forman (1552–1611), John Lambe (1545/6–1628), whom Poeton refers to, and Richard Napier (1559–1634). They were popular, and despite the borderline illegality of their practices, many people made use of them, and there was very little interest in bringing them to trial. Napier, for example, whose services included exorcisms, the provision of amulets and charms, and the casting of horoscopes,

[32] See James Sharpe, "The Witch's Familiar in Elizabethan England" in G. W. Bernard and Steven J. Gunn, eds., *Authority and Consent in Tudor England: Essays Presented to C. S. L. Davies* (Aldershot: Ashgate, 2002); James A. Sherpell, "Guardian Spirits or Demonic Pets—The Concept of the Witch's Familiar in Early Modern England, 1530–1712," in Angela N. H. Creager and William Chester Jordan, eds., *The Animal/Human Boundary: Historical Perspectives* (Rochester, NY: University of Rochester Press, 2002); Orna Alyagon Darr, *Marks of an Absolute Witch—Evidentiary Dilemmas in Early Modern England* (Farnham: Ashgate, 2011), chap. 6.

[33] For the history of cunning folk, see Owen Davies, *Popular Magic—Cunning-folk in English History* (London: Hambledon Continuum, 2007), chap. 3; Willem de Blécourt, "Witch Doctors, Soothsayers and Priests. On Cunning Folk in European Historiography and Tradition," *Social History*, 19, 3 (1994): 285–303; Kirsteen Macpherson Bardell, "Beyond Pendle: the 'lost' Lancashire witches," in Robert Poole, ed., *The Lancashire Witches: Histories and Stories* (Manchester: Manchester University Press, 2002).

as well as more conventional medicine, had tens of thousands of patients and was well-respected in his day.[34] As already mentioned, interest in prosecuting people for witchcraft of any kind seems to have been waning even further than usual in the 1630s, particularly in official circles. Arminian Bishop Richard Mountague removed reference to popular magic from his 1634 articles of visitation for the diocese of Chichester (which included Petworth), as Dandridge points out, and it may have been partly in response to this that Poeton penned his treatise on the subject.[35]

Poeton takes his place in a long line of European authors, mostly clerics, who wrote in condemnation of popular magical practitioners, stretching back far into the medieval period.[36] His work should be read in this wider context, but more specifically in the context of the attacks in this vein that came from the English Puritans who wrote treatises on witchcraft in the late sixteenth and seventeenth centuries. Authors such as George Gifford, William Perkins, and Richard Bernard wrote books on the subject of witchcraft in which the primary target was not just the harmful witch of popular stereotype (both then and now) but the ostensibly beneficial white witch.[37] The common people's supposedly excessive concern with black witches and lack of concern about white witches was a common complaint of all these writers. The image of the tyrannical preacher stirring up the populace against witches is a myth; but where the clergy and their allies did call for much greater implementation of the law was against healing "witches," those who did good within the community. For obvious reasons, there was little popular appetite for prosecuting such figures, and the concerns of such authors appear to have been largely ignored.

[34] On Napier, see Michael MacDonald, *Mystical Bedlam: Madness, Anxiety, and Healing in Seventeenth-Century England* (Cambridge: Cambridge University Press, 1981); on Forman, see Lauren Kassell, *Medicine and Magic in Elizabethan London: Simon Forman—Astrologer, Alchemist, & Physician* (Oxford: Oxford University Press, 2005); on Lambe, see below, explanatory note 3. For a sixteenth-century case study, see Alec Ryrie, *The Sorcerer's Tale: Faith and Fraud in Tudor England* (Oxford: Oxford University Press, 2008).

[35] Dandridge, "Anti-Quack Literature," 207; for some statistics on witchcraft prosecution during this period, see Sharpe, *Instruments*, 108–10.

[36] For the long view, see Euan Cameron, *Enchanted Europe—Superstition, Reason, and Religion, 1250–1750* (Oxford: Oxford University Press, 2010); Michael D. Bailey, *Magic and Superstition in Europe—A Concise History from Antiquity to the Present* (Plymouth: Rowman & Littlefield Publishers, 2007). On demonology and its intellectual context during the early modern period in particular, see Stuart Clark, *Thinking With Demons: The Idea of Witchcraft in Early Modern Europe* (Oxford: Oxford University Press, 1997).

[37] See Clark, *Thinking With Demons*, chap. 31.

Poeton certainly knew Bernard's treatise, and he borrows and adapts material from it;[38] he may also have been familiar with Gifford's *Dialogve*, and though his reading in this area does not appear to have been large, his arguments are generally conventional. The main contention of the Puritan demonologists was that any supernatural act which did not have a clear divine sanction must come from the Devil, and therefore even white magic was diabolical, as it had no such sanction. By masquerading as good (and indeed as Christian), white magic was actually far more pernicious than black magic, as people were more likely to make use of it and thus, the argument ran, to be seduced to the Devil's party. Black witches merely harmed the body, but white witches harmed the soul. The Puritans in particular argued that as it was sin which caused misfortune (as punishment from divine providence or as a trial of faith), it was these sins which should be the focus of any response to bewitchment, rather than a rush to prosecute people as witches, and in this way their writings on witchcraft formed part of a much wider project of Puritan social reform. Poeton seems to have been a moderate Calvinist rather than a Puritan,[39] and his central concern in the *Winnowing* is with the role of the physician. His arguments were also part of a wider campaign, but it was against unorthodox medical practitioners rather than ungodly living, as we shall see.

Poeton's arguments largely turn on a question of definition: white witches, according to Poeton, were not widely considered to *be* witches (21)—hence their other names, such as wise men/women or cunning folk. It was only those who practiced harmful magic who were considered to be witches, and who were feared by ordinary people:

> in common account, none are reputed to be witches, but onely such who are thought to have both will and skill to hurt man and beast: but that any have power so to doe, by any association with, or assistance from Sathan (without divine permission) I utterly deny. For Sathan himself cannot hurt either man or beast, untill such time that hee hath obtayned licence thereto from the Almighty . . . Yet are these miserable miscreants hated by the moste, feared by some, fawned on by others: as if they lyved without the lists or lyberties, of divine power or providence. And on the contrary, the white witches they are admired, applauded, yea well nigh adored (by some of the sottish sorte). And by to many, countenanced, pleaded for and protected. (6-7)

[38] Bernard's work was also influential on the notorious East Anglian witch hunt of 1645–1647. John Stearne, partner of "Witchfinder General" Matthew Hopkins, plagiarised Bernard's treatise heavily in his 1648 defense of the witch hunt; see Simon Davies, ed., *The Discovery of Witches and Witchcraft—The Writings of the Witchfinders* (Brighton: Puckrel Publishing, 2007). For Poeton's use of Bernard, see Appendix.

[39] Dandridge, "Anti-Quack Literature," 126.

The common argument is neatly expressed by Gregory: "zuch vokes as doo no harme, shud not bee witches" (34). People were perfectly familiar with the commandment, "Thou shalt not suffer a witch to live" (Exodus 22:18); the problem was they didn't think it applied to cunning folk. The root of this objection is that the Devil, being evil, can surely do no good, nor inspire anyone else so to do. This was a thorny problem for those of Poeton's stripe, who had to convince people that the Devil was perfectly capable of doing good in the short term in order to do harm in the long term: to help the body (not to mention the purse) at the expense of the soul. As Poeton puts it, "the devil will be very industrious to be an instrument of bodily health, either unto man or beaste, if in the interim; hee can (by any sleight or stratagem) wreake, hurt, or wounde the soule." (20) And damage to the soul was far more dangerous than anything minor like damage to bodily health or death, which was all that black witches could manage. The key scriptural support here is 2 Corinthians 11:14, "Satan himself is transformed into an angel of light," a verse to which Poeton returns throughout the treatise, and which was popular with demonologists. Satan performed his role as enemy of mankind not simply by killing people (though he might do this too, as long as God permitted), but far more widely and more perniciously, it was argued, by tempting people into sinful ways—and in order to do this, of course, he had to actually be tempting, rather than terrifying. As William Perkins, the leading English author in this respect, put it:

> For this must alwaies, be remembred, as a conclusion, that by Witches we vnderstand not those onely which kill and torment: but all Diuiners, Charmers, Iuglers, all Wizzards, commonly called wise men and wise women; yea, whosoeuer doe any thing (knowing what they doe) which cannot be effected by nature or art; and in the same number we reckon all good Witches, which doe no hurt but good, which doe not spoile and destroy, but saue and deliuer. All these come vnder this sentence of *Moses* [i.e., Exodus 22:18], because they deny God, and are confederates with Satan.[40]

This statement also includes another element of the argument, which was that, never mind the false benefits of their effects, the practices of white witches alone made them diabolical, and fit to be termed witches. Poeton's divine is at pains to convince Gregory of this fact: "For if they learne and practice, those thinges of the which the devill was the first inventor: I then see nothing to the contrary, but that they may justly be denominated his disciples." (72) Unlearned healing and the misuse of prayer needed to be recognized for what they were: not merely harmless error but the work of Satan.

[40] William Perkins, *A Discovrse Of The Damned Art of Witchcraft* (Cambridge: Cantrell Legge, 1608), 255–56.

Although many of Poeton's arguments are put into the mouth of a divine, his theological case largely consists of citation of scriptural examples, and his engagement with divinity is far more superficial than that of his clerical co-polemicists. Where he is on much stronger ground—and, indeed, where his arguments are measurably more practical than those of the clerics—is on issues surrounding the practice of medicine. The other important context for Poeton's treatise, therefore, is the issue of medicine more widely and, more specifically, the attack by licensed medical practitioners on unlicensed and unlearned medical practitioners, which came into full swing in the first half of the seventeenth century. While white witches made up a large proportion of this category of people, it also included a range of other figures such as empirics and priest-physicians, figures which Poeton also includes in his broad-church definition of "white witches."

Licensed medical practitioners included physicians, such as Poeton, as well as surgeons, apothecaries, and midwives. Of these, physicians were generally of the highest economic and social status. Physicians were, in general, responsible for diagnosing and curing internal maladies, while surgeons dealt with external injuries and conditions. Apothecaries prepared medical remedies, ostensibly at the direction of physicians and surgeons, though they were often sought out for and gave medical advice in their own right. Midwives, of course, dealt with childbirth.[41] As already discussed, Poeton described himself as "Licentiate in Physick and Chyrurgery" (surgery). Physicians could obtain a license to practice from bishops, from the universities, and from the Royal College of Physicians of London. Poeton appears to have had only an Episcopal license; this may have been part of his reason for moving out of London, where the approval of the College would have been required in order for him to practice.[42] Importantly, whether or not they had attended university and whether or not they were licensed by the Royal College (as the majority were not), all the various types of licensed physician "considered themselves learned and opposed the multitude of unlearned practitioners."[43]

The vast majority of those who practiced medicine during this period, however, "did so without the blessing of church, state or occupational organization."[44]

---

41 See Beier, *Sufferers and Healers*, chap. 2. On the history of medicine during the period, see also: Roger French and Andrew Wear, eds., *The Medical Revolution of the Seventeenth Century* (Cambridge: Cambridge University Press, 1989); Ian Mortimer, *The Dying and the Doctors: The Medical Revolution in Seventeenth-Century England* (London: Royal Historical Society, 2009); Mary Lindemann, *Medicine and Society in Early Modern Europe* (Cambridge: Cambridge University Press, 2010).

42 Dandridge, "Anti-Quack Literature," 120.

43 Beier, *Sufferers and Healers*, 11. See also Margaret Pelling, *Medical Conflicts in Early Modern London: Patronage, Physicians, and Irregular Practitioners, 1550–1640* (Oxford: Oxford University Press, 2003).

44 Beier, *Sufferers and Healers*, 19.

Their number included white witches properly so called, but also quacks, herbalists, and empirics. Empirics were those who, as their name suggests, considered that practical experience to be of greater value than theoretical education; they were anti-intellectual, and although their methods may have obtained results, it is easy to see how their ideas undermined the status of traditionally-educated physicians.[45] Also included were the moonlighters known as priest-physicians. Ross Dandridge argues that the *Winnowing*, following on from the *Vrinall*, is in large part concerned with priest-physicians—clergymen who also practiced medicine—in particular. This is evidenced primarily, Dandridge argues, by Poeton's repeated return to the issue of uroscopy throughout the treatise, an issue of little concern to other writers against white witches but which, as Poeton made clear in the *Vrinall*, was a widespread practice among priest-physicians (though it was also in common use by empirics).[46] A primary argument against priest-physicians was the inappropriateness of divines meddling in physical matters, or of physicians meddling in matters of the spirit.[47] Poeton embodies his objection to this professional interdisciplinarity in the very structure of his treatise, with separate characters (a divine and a physician) introduced to deal with their separate specialisms. Priest-physicians also had a tendency to favor occult means such as charms and blessings in their cures in a manner considered by their opponents to be papist, if not downright Satanic.

A particularly pernicious practice of unlicensed healers (as Poeton saw it) was uroscopy: the diagnosis of illness via examination of the patient's urine. As we have already seen, Poeton had written an entire treatise dedicated to the topic, now bound with the *Winnowing*. He returns to the subject throughout the *Winnowing*, and it was clearly still heavily on his mind. James Hart, who in the 1620s also wrote a treatise against the practice, claimed that uroscopy was "growne now adayes a common custome."[48] It certainly seems to have been a popular service, frequently requested by clients, and indeed even many physicians had no qualms about offering it. In the *Winnowing* Poeton develops his arguments on the practice to an extreme—not only is it erroneous and the result of poor education, uromancy is actually diabolical. It "can no way be performed by lawfull art," he writes (38), and skill in diagnosing from urine is among the diabolically-received powers of the two occultists who attempt to seduce Poeton to their side; of all their unholy knowledge, "This of all the rest seemed moste strange unto mee," he states (45), and later reveals that their skill therein was the result of aid from

[45] See Beier, *Sufferers and Healers*, 20–23.

[46] Dandridge, "Anti-Quack Literature," 182–83.

[47] See David Harley, "James Hart of Northampton and the Calvinist Critique of Priest-Physicians: An Unpublished Polemic of the Early 1620s," *Medical History*, 42 (1998): 362–86, for a good discussion of this issue, as well as an edition of a contemporary treatise on the subject.

[48] Hart, *Anatomie of Vrines*, 12.

the wicked spirits they summoned in the guise of angels (53). It is listed among the powers promised by the Devil to those he is seeking to tempt (62). Poeton was vehemently opposed to the practice of uroscopy, and was clearly determined to eradicate it by any means necessary. In many ways the *Winnowing* should be considered a further entry into the seventeenth-century controversy over the "Uromantike art" (16).

A further type of unorthodox healer in the period were those who healed by touch, often known as "strokers," and the Boy of Godlyman, whom Poeton discusses at the end of his treatise, is an example of one of these. The Boy (or "Prophet") of Godlyman (i.e., Godalming, in Surrey, not far north of Petworth) is a seventh son, a feature which was typical of such people. Healing by touch was a power claimed by a number of monarchs, notably the Stuarts, it must be recalled, so belief in its virtue went to the very top of society. Poeton appears to be the only source for this particular figure, who was apparently popular and who is said to have cured a woman with a facial ulcer (who it seems Poeton himself had talked to). There is evidence of a number of figures very similar to the Boy of Godlyman from throughout the seventeenth century, however, so the case was not unusual.[49] The most well-known of these is Valentine Greatrakes (1629–1683), an Irish stroker whose visit to England in 1666 brought him widespread fame and notoriety and saw him summoned to meet Charles II, which inspired a brief print controversy.[50] Poeton's argument in respect of the Boy of Godlyman's apparent powers is that, seeing as miracles are no longer an active force in the world and therefore there can be no divine warrant for his abilities, they must, it follows, be diabolical. As with white witches, any sort of supernatural ability which did not have orthodox scriptural support was condemned by the educated as Satanic. Poeton's response is careful and measured, however, and he goes into some detail, perhaps because of the delicate nature of this area (given that Stuart kings claimed the power of healing by touch).

Throughout the treatise, Poeton in fact tends to blur all the boundaries between the different types of unlicensed and unlearned healers. However, so did their clients—those in need of medical assistance would have drawn no distinction, not only between types of unlicensed healers but between licensed and unlicensed healers as well. They were, understandably, more concerned with results than anything else. The popular concern with results over education or divine sanction was a persistent complaint of those who attacked the existence of unlicensed healers, just as it was for those who attacked the existence of cunning

[49] See Thomas, *Religion and the Decline of Magic*, 236–42, esp. 239; Beier, *Sufferers and Healers*, 25–26; and for the wider geographical and chronological context, see Stephen Wilson, *The Magical Universe: Everyday Ritual and Magic in Pre-Modern Europe* (London and New York: Hambledon and London, 2000), chap. 13.

[50] See Peter Elmer, *The Miraculous Conformist: Valentine Greatrakes, the Body Politic and the Politics of Healing in Post Restoration Britain* (Oxford: Oxford University Press, 2012).

folk and termed them witches. In any case, the boundaries between the different types of practitioners were genuinely blurred in reality—not least because different types of practitioner, whether learned or unlearned, very often shared the same medical techniques and remedies.[51] Although there may have been a preponderance of, say, charms and spells among cunning folk, for instance, they should not be considered solely occult practitioners only interested in spirits and magic books; many of the remedies they offered would have been little different from those offered by apothecaries or licensed physicians.

Unlicensed and unlearned practitioners were the target of repeated attacks from licensed physicians, in large part because they represented both a commercial and an ideological threat. A notable predecessor to Poeton is John Cotta, in whose work *A Short Discoverie Of The Vnobserved Dangers of seuerall sorts of ignorant and vnconsiderate Practisers of Physicke* the links with witchcraft are also made explicit, and whose arguments are often very similar to Poeton's. Cotta is particularly notable because he went on to publish a treatise entirely dedicated to the subject of witchcraft, in which he reiterates the attack on quack healers. In both works Cotta foreshadows Poeton's arguments about the importance of using the services of educated physicians (and the dangers of not doing so).[52] The very existence of unlicensed practitioners cast doubt on the validity of the years of academic training the Royal College of Physicians required for its members. And as they were invariably cheaper than licensed practitioners, the latter being beyond the means of many people, they were often a popular choice for those in need of medical assistance. The authors who attacked them consistently complained about the way in which such figures were considered a legitimate alternative to the services of licensed physicians. Poeton's tract should be read partly in the context of this effort on behalf of licensed physicians both to bolster the reputation and standing of their own craft and to discredit the multitude of unlicensed and unlearned healers.[53] Not only was their long training and extensive experience essential to the diagnosing and curing of illness, physicians were appointed by God and sanctioned by scripture—practicing medicine without it was impi-

---

[51] See Beier, *Sufferers and Healers*, 31.

[52] John Cotta, *A Short Discoverie Of The Vnobserved Dangers of seuerall sorts of ignorant and vnconsiderate Practisers of Physicke in England* (London: for William Jones and Richard Boyle, 1612) and *The Infallible Trve And Assvred Witch* (London: John Legate for Richard Higgenbotham, 1624) (this is the second, revised and expanded, edition of his *Triall of Witch-craft*, originally published in 1616). Similar attacks on quack healers which were published in print include: Johann Oberndorff and Francis Herring, *The Anatomyes of the True Physition* (London: for Arthur Johnson, 1602); James Hart, *The Diet of The Diseased* (London: John Beale for Robert Allot, 1633); James Primerose, *Popular Errours. Or The Errours of the People In Physick*, trans. Robert Wittie (London: W. Wilson for Nicholas Bourne, 1651).

[53] See Beier, *Sufferers and Healers*, chap. 2; Dandridge, "Anti-Quack Literature."

ous as well as dangerous. In the *Winnowing* Poeton regularly returns to the issue of the lack of education on the part of white witches and the implausibility of their effecting successful cures as a result. Indeed, such was the unlikeliness of someone with no standard medical education becoming a successful healer, he argues, that if cures from such people *were* seen to be effective, there must be some diabolical supernatural assistance lying behind. The stakes were much higher than simple commercial competition, therefore: this was also a battle for people's souls.

Another practice whose boundaries blur into those discussed here, and which also comes under Poeton's censure, is scholarly ritual magic. Widely practiced in the medieval period, ritual magic was largely diminishing as a scholarly pursuit by the seventeenth century, but there were still many who took an interest in the area.[54] Indeed, ritual magic may actually have been more widely practiced during the period than we realize, and evidence such as Poeton offers here seems to support this suggestion. Poeton recounts the story (in the guise of the physician character in the dialogue, but the story is marked in the margin as "Thauthors free confession") of two men, one a dissolute libertine and the other a strict ascetic, who together allegedly attempted to introduce the young Poeton to the practice of ritual magic. The ostensible aim was for Poeton, who was not, he writes, enamored of extensive study, to take an easy route to knowledge and to success as a physician. Sadly it seems unlikely that we will be able to identify these two men, assuming the narrative to be true. The odd parallelism of their offers (44) seems implausible, although the seven years they each ask Poeton to live with them may be a reflection of the typical length of an apprenticeship. The knowledge of the black arts that the narrator recounts at least has the ring of truth, reflecting as it does known practices far more widely, and whether or not the details are true, the story is surely based on Poeton's own knowledge to some degree. It is a fascinating insight into the world of this kind of magic, which has left so few traces from the period. Though his story is by far the most detailed, Poeton was not alone among writers on witchcraft to have dabbled in his youth—Thomas Cooper, author of *The Mystery Of Witch craft* (1617), tells a very similar story of his university days, and even William Perkins was a devotee of

[54] On the history of ritual magic, see: P. G. Maxwell-Stuart, *Wizards: A History* (Stroud: Tempus, 2004); Clark, *Thinking With Demons*, chaps. 14 and 15; Bengkt Ankarloo, Stuart Clark, and William Monter, *Witchcraft and Magic in Europe: The Period of the Witch Trials* (Philadelphia: University of Pennsylvania Press, 2002), pt. 3, chap. 3; Frank Klaassen, *The Transformations of Magic: Illicit Learned Magic in the Later Middle Ages and Renaissance* (University Park: Pennsylvania State University Press, 2013); Richard Kieckhefer, *Magic in the Middle Ages* (Cambridge: Cambridge University Press, 1987); Brian Vickers, ed., *Occult & Scientific Mentalities in the Renaissance* (Cambridge: Cambridge University Press, 1984); and below, nn. 56 and 57.

astrology when he was young.[55] Particularly notable in Poeton's case is the strong link between magic and the practice of medicine—the purpose of their magical powers being to increase the magus's skill as a physician.

The specific type of ritual magic that the two men in Poeton's narrative practice is perhaps the most common kind, and abundant evidence survives for the medieval period in particular of this kind of ritual. The two men summon spirits, whom they believe to be angels, in the hope of obtaining from them knowledge and power. Belief in the possibility of invoking and conversing with angels was relatively widespread in early modern Europe; it was fundamental to the philosophy of Neoplatonism. And while many, like Poeton, condemned it as impious and diabolical (the spirits were not angels, they said, but devils in disguise), there were also many who believed the angels to be genuine and the process both a holy and an orthodox one. Magic was always a contested category—angelic ritual magic had regularly been condemned as unholy by theologians, even while its practitioners claimed it as a high form of devotion.[56] A number of manuscripts survive with examples of ritual invocations aimed at summoning angels; these kind of grimoires are presumably along the same lines as the Vocabula mentioned by Poeton.[57]

---

55 Thomas Cooper, *The Mystery Of Witch-craft* (London: Nicholas Okes, 1617), 9–13; William Perkins, *Fovre Great Lyers* (London: Robert Waldegrave, 1585), B1ʳ.

56 On angels in the period, see: Peter Marshall and Alexandra Walsham, eds., *Angels in the Early Modern World* (Cambridge: Cambridge University Press, 2006); Joad Raymond, *Milton's Angels: The Early-Modern Imagination* (Oxford: Oxford University Press, 2010); idem, ed., *Conversations with Angels: Towards a History of Spiritual Communication, 1100–1700* (Basingstoke: Palgrave Macmillan, 2011); Laura Sangha, *Angels and Belief in England, 1480–1700* (London: Pickering & Chatto, 2012); Clare Copeland and Jan Machielsen, eds., *Angels of Light? Sanctity and the Discernment of Spirits in the Early Modern Period* (Leiden: Brill, 2013). For the medieval background, see Claire Fanger, ed., *Conjuring Spirits: Texts and Traditions of Medieval Ritual Magic* (University Park: Pennsylvania State University Press, 1998).

57 For some accessible examples of instructions for angelic ritual magic, see: Adam McLean, ed., *A Treatise on Angel Magic: Being a Complete Transcription of Ms. Harley 6482 in the British Library* (Grand Rapids: Phanes Press, 1990), an example of a mid-seventeenth century treatise on angel magic, including instructions for invoking angelic spirits and how to determine good angels from bad (an issue which crops up in Poeton's treatise); Folger Shakespeare Library MS V.b.26 (1), available online at http://luna.folger.edu/luna/servlet/s/472uem; bk. 15 in Reginald Scot, *The discouerie of witchcraft* (London: [Henry Denham for] William Brome, 1584), and bk. 15, chap. 7, in the 1665 edition of Scot's treatise, part of the anonymous additions to this edition (London: for Andrew Clark to be sold by Dixy Page, 1665); *Henry Cornelius Agrippa his Fourth Book Of Occult Philosophy*, trans. Robert Turner (London: J. C. for John Harrison, 1655); *Ars Notoria: The Notory Art Of Solomon*, trans. Robert Turner (London: J. Cottrel to be sold by Martha Harrison, 1657).

The most famous example of a practitioner of angel magic is John Dee (1527–1609), the mathematician, astrologer, and magus, who spent many years (so he believed) in conversation with angels. An edition of Dee's diaries of his angelic conversations was published by Meric Casaubon (who would later write treatises in favor of belief in witchcraft) in 1659, as *A True & Faithful Relation Of What passed for many Yeers Between Dr. John Dee (A Mathematician of Great Fame in Q. Eliz. and King James their Reignes) and Some Spirits*; it is the most extensive account of angelic interaction to have survived from the period.[58] Casaubon believed the conversations to be real, but with fallen angels (i.e., devils); the work was published in order to counteract what Casaubon saw as a growing disbelief in spirits and spiritual interaction, which in turn, Casaubon and others like him worried, was a high road to atheism. While there were many who criticized Dee in his own day, there were many others who echoed his beliefs. Dee's biographer Glyn Parry demonstrates that, far from being fringe ideas, such beliefs were thoroughly integrated at the very highest levels of Elizabethan society. Richard Napier, who has already been mentioned, practiced angel magic, very much in the vein of Dee (in fact Napier had met Dee early in the century).[59] Astrologer William Lilly also dabbled in the area.[60] Far from disappearing from view as the century progressed, there was a growing interest in angel magic in the early 1640s, as Joad Raymond has demonstrated.[61] Poeton's treatise provides further evidence of the prevalence of such beliefs, and makes clear once again the decidedly blurred boundaries between types of magic and types of magical practitioner.

Related to these discussions of the boundaries of medicine and magic is a topical subject that Poeton briefly touches on at the end of his treatise: the weapon-salve. A form of sympathetic magic, the weapon-salve had been the subject of a recent minor print controversy in England. Richard Bernard defines it as "The healing of a wound by anoynting the instrument which gaue the wound."[62] The weapon which had caused the wound in question was treated with a rather gruesome concoction, while still stained with the victim's blood, and by a form of sympathetic attraction this contributed to the wound's recovery. The controversy had begun in England in 1631, with the publication by Buckinghamshire clergyman William Foster of *Hoplocrismaspongvs: Or, A Sponge to wipe away the Weapon-Salve.*[63] The ground of Foster's attack was not that the weapon-salve did not work, but that it was diabolical in nature: tantamount to witchcraft. The

[58] (London: D. Maxwell for T. Garthwait, 1659).

[59] MacDonald, *Mystical Bedlam*, 16–19. MacDonald perhaps overstates the level of opposition to such magic amongst those Protestants not of the Puritan bent.

[60] Raymond, *Milton's Angels*, 106–11.

[61] Raymond, *Milton's Angels*, chap. 4.

[62] Richard Bernard, *A Gvide To Grand-Ivry Men* (London: Felix Kingston for Edward Blackmore, 1627), 125.

[63] (London: Thomas Cotes for John Grove, 1631).

invention of the cure was ascribed by Foster, as it was by many (though erroneously), to German physician and occultist Paracelsus, who had a large following in England, and who was himself accused by Foster of being a witch.[64] Poeton had read Foster's tract and was in agreement with him.

Foster's sponge was targeted primarily at renowned physician Robert Fludd—Foster went so far as to have a copy of the title page of his tract nailed to Fludd's front door—and Fludd published a very swift and detailed response, also in 1631, and which Poeton had also read. Fludd's tract argued for the natural efficacy of the cure and sought to repudiate the accusation that it involved supernatural agency.[65] Fludd was a respected member of the Royal College of Physicians, which may explain why Poeton is unwilling to criticize him too fiercely. Fludd's support for the belief demonstrates that it was not an idea from the outer margins of early modern culture, but a serious remedy investigated and maintained by educated men. Interestingly, part of Fludd's response to Foster involved criticizing the latter's lack of learning, which was exactly the accusation Poeton and others levelled at unlicensed medical practitioners.[66] Widespread interest in the cure is demonstrated by the success of a defense of it published by Sir Kenelm Digby in the 1650s, which ran into numerous editions.[67]

That the weapon-salve was still a pressing issue at this time is demonstrated by the very fact that Poeton felt the need to address it. Poeton acknowledges his own lack of knowledge in respect of the salve, and somewhat tentatively advances his opinion that "the devill hath a finger, if not a hand therein." (64) Relying on Foster and Bernard, Poeton argues that if the creators of the weapon-salve were witches, then the salve itself can hardly be wholesome. Poeton only briefly criticizes Fludd, but it is clear where his sympathies lie in this respect. It is important to recognize that his assessment is based on a relatively open-minded assessment

[64] See Allen G. Debus, "Robert Fludd and the Use of Gilbert's *De Magnete* in the Weapon-Salve Controversy," *Journal of the History of Medicine and Allied Sciences*, 19, 4 (1964): 389–417; idem, *The Chemical Philosophy: Paracelsian Science and Medicine in the Sixteenth and Seventeenth Centuries*, 2 vols. (New York: Science History Pub., 1977), I, 279–90; Lauren Kassell, "Magic, Alchemy and the Medical Economy in Early Modern England: The Case of Robert Fludd's Magnetical Medicine," in Mark S. R. Jenner and Patrick Wallis, eds., *Medicine and the Market in England and Its Colonies, c. 1450–c. 1850* (Basingstoke: Palgrave Macmillan, 2007).

[65] Robert Fludd, *Doctor Flvdds Answer unto M. Foster Or, The Sqvesing Of Parson Fosters Sponge, ordained by him for the wiping away of the Weapon-Salve* (London: for Nathaniel Butter, 1631). Fludd had mentioned his belief in the weapon-salve in his earlier work, *Anatomiae amphitheatrum* (Frankfurt, 1623); see Debus, "Robert Fludd," 393.

[66] Fludd, *Doctor Flvdds Answer unto M. Foster*, A3^r^.

[67] Kenelm Digby, *A Late Discourse . . . Touching the Cure of Wounds by the Powder of Sympathy*, trans. R. White (London: R. Lowndes and T. Davies, 1658). See Thomas, *Religion and the Decline of Magic*, 225.

of the facts, however, as with his discussion of the Boy of Godlyman, rather than mere dogmatism.

This Edition: Editorial Procedures

As discussed above, Poeton's treatise survives in a single fair copy, almost certainly in Poeton's own hand; therefore it presents almost no textual difficulty. The intention in this edition has been to strike a balance between readability and fidelity to Poeton's writing. In general the editorial approach has been conservative. Poeton's original spelling, punctuation, and capitalization have been retained, with the following exceptions:

Where usage of u/v and i/j is not in accordance with modern practice, it has been modernized. Poeton, however, in a manner typical of the (in this respect) transitional period in which he was writing, is often in accordance with modern practice in any case; that is, although there are a few consonantal "u"s, he very often uses "v"s, as in modern practice. For the sake of readability, therefore, his usage has been regularized. A somewhat serious problem which follows on from this occurs with Gregory's dialect form of "devil," "dule." Modernizing this to "dvle" looks very clumsy, but it is unlikely that the intended pronunciation is "dool" or "duel." Some form of pronunciation along the lines of "duvvel" is presumably intended. To solve the problem, an apostrophe has been inserted to make "d'vle," with the hope of more accurately reflecting the intended pronunciation. This form has the virtue of being closer to the modern "devil," which it is intended to represent. Other features of secretary hand, such as the long "s" or the dot which Poeton (very considerately) adds under a medial "u" in order to distinguish it from an "n," have not been reproduced.

Capitalization of proper nouns has been silently regularized. Poeton switches between capitals both for books of scripture and for names without apparent logic; in any case, with some of Poeton's letter forms it is not entirely clear if capitalization is intended. Capitalization has also been introduced at the beginning of sentences, where it is missing, in order to aid comprehension. Otherwise Poeton's original capitalization, along with its irregularities, has been retained.

Contractions and abbreviations, with the exception of the ampersand, have been silently expanded. Poeton usually abbreviates the titles of books of scripture, for example; these have been expanded to aid the reader; the full stop or colon used after the title of the book has been removed (Poeton uses these even when the titles are not abbreviated, but this has not been reproduced). In some cases this has meant modernizing the name of the book in question (e.g., with Jeremiah or Deuteronomy), but this has been felt to be unavoidable, and in any case Poeton is not consistent in his spelling in this respect. There are a number of further exceptions to this practice: where "verse" and "chapter" are abbreviated in references, it was felt that expansion would unnecessarily clutter the text and, as the sense is self-evident, they have been left abbreviated; "Dr," "Mr" and "viz." have not been expanded, given that they will be familiar to modern readers (although it should be noted that "Mr" is a contraction of "master" rather than "mister"); and finally Poeton uses "saint," "Saint" and "S^{t}" indistinguishably—these have been regularized to "St" in references and titles and expanded elsewhere. In cases where it is required, the abbreviation mark has been regularized to a full stop (Poeton often uses a colon) and removed where it would not occur in modern usage (e.g., with "Dr"). When a dash over a medial letter is used to indicate a contraction of a letter that would be superfluous in modern spelling (e.g., a second "n" in "sin"), the extra letter has not been added and the contraction has been ignored (given that Poeton's spelling of such words varies in any case).

Punctuation, with the exceptions already noted, has been retained as in the original. This may lead to some difficulties for modern readers, given Poeton's liberal use of the colon and semi-colon where we would use commas, but it retains the flavor of his writing and is easy enough once one gets used to it. Instances in which Poeton uses a full stop for a comma, however, have been amended in order to aid comprehension. A further exception here is the virgule, which Poeton uses as a form of "hard" full stop (he often uses a full stop alone where we would use a comma or a colon); the virgule has been removed and capitalization (as explained above) introduced where it was lacking to aid the sense in such instances. Full stops placed within or before brackets have been placed outside and behind where necessary.

There are a number of corrections and insertions throughout the manuscript; however, it is a fair copy, and the vast majority, if not all, of these are errors made (presumably) in transcription and corrected either as the manuscript was written or on a later read through. Erasures have therefore not been reproduced. Insertions have been silently inserted in the appropriate place; it has not been considered necessary to mark them as the majority are simply basic transcription errors, without which the text would not make sense. Where they have been thought to contain potential significance, they are mentioned in the explanatory notes. Other obvious errors have been silently corrected (e.g., "dwone" for "downe"), but there are very few of these, and where there is any doubt they have been left untouched. Incorrect scriptural references have been silently corrected (again, there are very few). Parentheses left open have been closed in the most likely place.

Spacing has been regularized except in instances where Poeton clearly intended large spaces to be left within a line. The lineation of the original has not been retained, and the dashes used to fill up space at the end of lines have been omitted. Indentations have been added at the beginning of paragraphs.

Poeton's use of italics has been retained, replete with irregularity. It is clear that he placed some importance on this, given that on occasion he corrects himself when a word is begun in secretary hand which was intended to be in italic (e.g., in a quotation), though in many instances (such as with proper nouns) he is irregular in his application of the italic hand. The exception here is the occasional errors Poeton makes—for instance, writing an odd italic "h" in the middle of a word otherwise in secretary hand—these have been amended. Poeton's insertions are occasionally italicized, but this seems almost certainly to be incidental, therefore this has not been reproduced or signaled here. (It may perhaps indicate insertions made at a different time to the original writing of the manuscript, but there are no instances in which the sense is affected; they are merely errors.) Marginal notes in the original are in italic hand: this has been retained here. Poeton's two prefaces are also in italic in the original, but this has not been reproduced. Where he quotes Latin in the prefaces it has been given in italics, in accordance with his practice in the rest of the treatise, but other potential usages (e.g., names of scriptural books) have not been introduced. In any case, the boundaries between the two hands are blurred, and there are many shared letter forms between the two. Poeton was writing at an age when secretary hand was gradually fading from use in favor of italic, and the indistinct boundary between the two hands in his own usage of them reflects this wider shift.

Once the above changes have been made, the text is in general straightforward to read, and it has not been deemed necessary to patronize the reader by making more sweeping modernizations, which would run the risk of losing the flavor and personality of the original. On the other side of the question, a fully diplomatic transcription was considered an excess; those who wish to experience the original exactly as it was may do so freely in the British Library. The original paper, ink, and handwriting are inextricable aspects of this experience.

Poeton's original page numbers are given in square brackets throughout, in order to allow the reader to collate this edition with the original manuscript.

Finally, as well as Poeton's own marginal notes, the treatise is annotated in the margin throughout in a second hand. These notes are not by Poeton and therefore have not been included in this edition. While this may smack of overzealous intentionalism, the secondary annotations seem to be more akin to annotations in a printed book, which would rarely be included in a modern edition of that book. See the discussion above for a more detailed consideration of these notes and the reasons against including them in this edition. Where it has been felt that the secondary annotator adds material to the work which is of potential significance or interest, their comments have been noted in the explanatory notes.

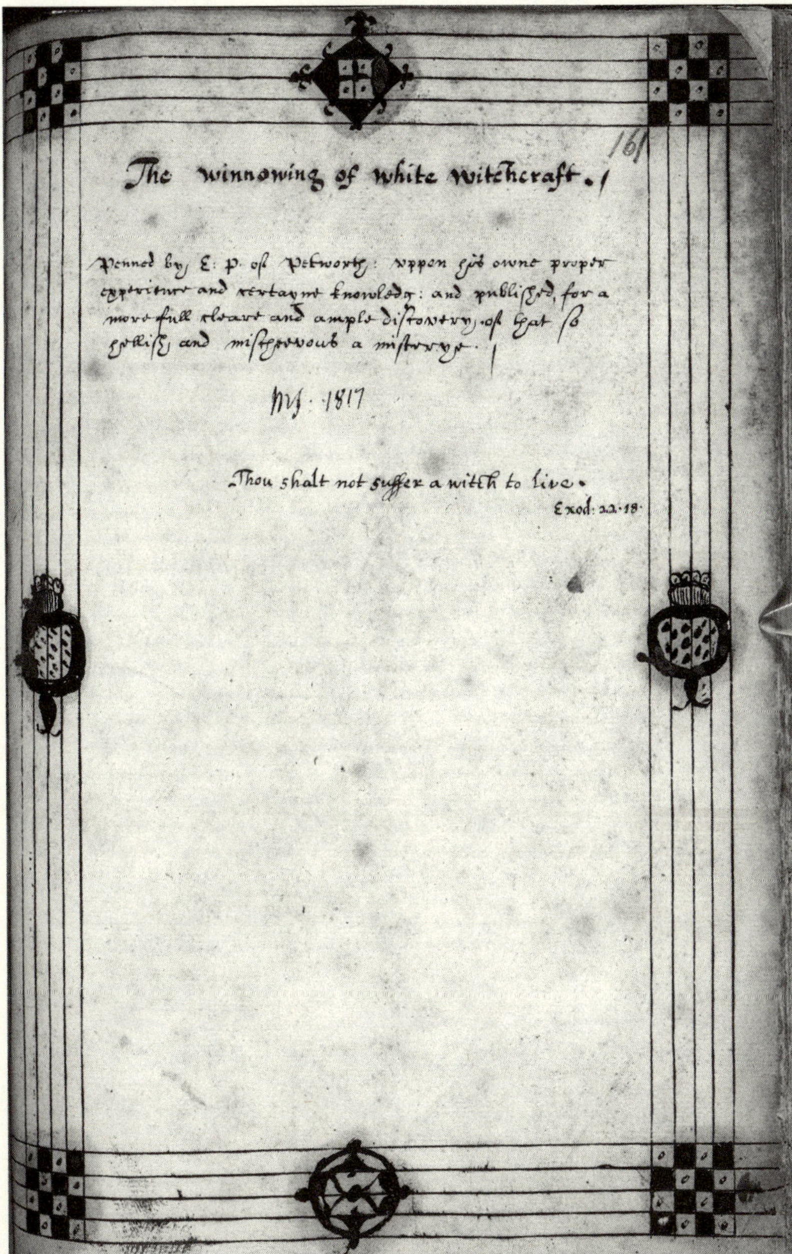

161

The winnowing of white witchcraft.

Penned by E: P. of Petworth: uppon his owne proper experience and certayne knowledge: and published, for a more full cleare and ample discovery, of that so hellish and mischevous a misterye.

Ms. 1817

Thou shalt not suffer a witch to live.
Exod: 22.18.

Fig 2: Title Page of *The Winnowing of White Wichcraft* © The British Library Board (Sloane MS 1954, fol. 161r).

[¶1]

The Winnowing of White Witchcraft.

Penned by E. P. of Petworth: uppon his owne proper experience and certayne knowledg: and published, for a more full cleare and ample discovery of that so hellish and mischeavous a misterye.

Thou shalt not suffer a witch to live.
Exodus 22. 18.

[¶1v blank]

[¶2]

To the right worshipful (and his much honoured frend) Sir Henry Dawtry (of Moore, in the parrish of Petworth, and County of Sussex) Knight, E. P. of Petworth, wisheth, internall peace: externall prosperity: and eternall felicitie.[1]

Right worshipful:

As you are the ancientest of all myne acquaintance in all these Southern parts: so have you ever (since I first knew you) been a moste loving, and kinde frend, both to my self and mine. In regard wherof, I do (and ever shall) both cheerfully and thankfully acknowledg the same. And shall ever be ready to express my thankfullnes towards your worthy self, that vertuous Lady your wife, and all yours. Sir: I know that God hath geven you a large hart in wisdome and understanding: enabling you to discerne twixt good and evill: and to put a difference, between the cleane and the uncleane, the pretious and the vile. Which hath emboldened mee (so much the rather) to lay this poore naked abortive labour of myne, at the gates of your loving acceptance, praying you to geve it entertaynment: though not for its merit, yet for the love of him, who devotes himself, and dedicates theis his poore labours unto the perpetuall honour of your ancient renowned name, whose vertues, promise a hopefull harvest of great encrease, both in your person and posterity. Right worthy Sir: you well know that our gracious God, accepted of goates hayre offerred unto him by the poore (for the use of his Tabernacle) as well as hee did of the goulde which was presented unto him by the rich. Exodus 25. 4. And our blessed saviour preferd the two Mites of the poore widdow, before the large bounty of such as had aboundance. Mark 12. 42. &c. Now knowing that you desyre to imitate God in all gracious disposition I commend this poore Orphan unto your prudent protection.

Humbly taking my leave. I rest

At your worships Command: in all respective dutyes of love and service during life.

Edward Poeton.

---

[1] As pointed out by Ross Dandridge, Henry Dawtry "was a member of one of Petworth's two leading gentry families, holding extensive land in both Sussex and Essex." "Anti-Quack Literature," 120.

[¶2v]

To the Christian reader.

Beloved:

I am verily perswaded that you are not ignorant of that precept of the moste high and moste holy God. Exodus 22. 18. Thou shalt not suffer a witch to lyve. And to the end that the people of God mought know who were witches, it pleased the lord: Leviticus 20. at ver. 27. to declare his sacred minde, in this matter, saying: A man or woman that hath a familiar spirit, or that is a wizard: shall surely be put to death: they shall stone them with stones &c.[2] Loe heer a moste cleare manifestation of the minde and judgement of the moste wise, moste high, and moste holy God. Which is so playne and perspicuous, that none (unles they be wilfully blinde) can pretend ignorance heerin. But alas; all this notwithstanding wee finde not, that among those many Judges, and Kings of Israell there was not any one (that is mentioned in holy writt) who executed that judgment of the almighty uppon those abhominable sinners: King Saul except: of whose act therein; wee finde som mention to be made. 1. Samuel 28. 9. Yet this King clave not stedfastly unto that law of the lord with a perfect hart, but did apostate therefrom; for he himselfe (in the depth of his distress) forsooke the lord: and went unto a witch at Endor to consult with her, as is to be seen in the last recited scripture, at ver. 7. And among all the kings of Judah, I reade not of any one, who did unto those who had famylyar spirits, and unto the wizards &c. performing the words of the law: good King Josiah except, of whose worthy acts therein, there remayneth a sacred recorde even unto this day. 2. Kings 23. ver. 24. Now although that it be most evident in sacred writt, that Witches, wizards, and such like cappitall offenders, are an abhomination unto the lord, as is moste apparant. Deuteronomy 18. ver. 10. 11. 12. yet as wee have seen they were not sought out and punished, (by the Judges and Kings of Israell and Judah) except before excepted. But on the contrary some of those greate ones favoured, countenanced, yea sought unto them, and consulted with them: yea and which was far worse gave themselves unto the practice of those abhominable infernall arts: as did King Manasseh. 2. Chronicles 33. ver. 6. As also Queen Jesabell. 2. Kings 9. ver. 22. So then, these things considered: it is not to be held a thing to be either new or strange, that white witches shoulde finde so

[2] Poeton uses the 1611 "Authorized" translation of the Bible.

many frends and favourers (as now they doe) in this last corrupt age of the world, in the which, moste men minde earthly thinges. **[¶3]** Alas: is it not much to be lamented to consider how many frends and favourers, that late lewde man (who was intiteled) Dr Lamb founde: Oh, was hee not resorted unto (and consulted with) by many persons, of no meane esteem in this world: yet was hee none other then a very witch. But lett us not forgett Gods just judgment uppon him in his end.[3] But woe and alas, lamentable it is to see, how the giddy headed vulgar, are affected to such kinde of peeple, as profess the Curing of witchcraft, the return of things stoln or strayed, to gether with the manifesting of all malladyes, belonging unto man, uppon the bare inspection of a carryed urine: which is a thing by any lawfull art unpossible to be effected. Which pointe I have sufficiently proved in another tract called the unmasking of urines uncertaynties.[4] But this I know, that in common account, none are reputed to be witches, but onely such who are thought to have both will and skill to hurt man and beast: but that any have power so to doe, by any association with, or assistance from

[3] John Lambe, astrologer and cunning man, was connected with George Villiers, the unpopular Duke of Buckingham, and Villiers may be among those Poeton has in mind here when he mentions persons "of no meane esteem in this world." Lambe was highly unpopular in London in his own right, and on 13 June 1628, after a visit to the Fortune Theatre, Lambe (then aged 82) was beaten to death by a mob. Ballads were written about his death, and an account of his alleged misdemeanours (which were not all related to the supernatural) was published shortly afterwards as *A Briefe Description Of The Notoriovs Life of Iohn Lambe, otherwise called Doctor Lambe. Together with his Ignominious Death* (Amsterdam [i.e., London: George Miller?] 1628). He had been accused of sorcery but the charges were dropped; he had also been accused of falsely claiming a license to practise medicine. In his defence of the latter, Lambe claimed that he only pretended to examine and treat people, in order to earn money. See Alastair Bellany, "The Murder of John Lambe: Crowd Violence, Court Scandal and Popular Politics in Early Seventeenth-Century England," *Past and Present*, 200 (2008): 37–76; Malcolm Gaskill, "Witchcraft, Politics, and Memory in Seventeenth-Century England," *The Historical Journal*, 50.2 (2007): 289–308; Anita McConnel, "Lambe, John (1545/6–1628)" in *ODNB*.

[4] Poeton will return to the issue of uromancy, or uroscopy—the diagnosis of illness via a visual examination of the patient's urine—throughout the treatise. As this comment indicates, he wrote a separate work dedicated to the subject, which is bound with the present treatise in Sloane MS 1954 (see introduction). It is not given the title used here, however (if this is indeed intended to be a title), which may indicate that it was written later than, or at least concurrently with, *The Winnowing*.

Sathan (without divine permission) I utterly deny. For Sathan himself cannot hurt either man or beast, untill such time that hee hath obtayned licence thereto from the Almighty: which is moste sounde and sure, as the worde of truthe testifieth unto us. As wee may see in the booke of Job chap. 1. &. 2. Agayne wee may reade. Matthew 8. Mark 5. & Luke 8. that the devill had not so much power as to prevayle over the swine of the Gadarens untill Christ licenced him thereto. For let us know (to our comfort) that Sathan is Gods slave, and that hee cannot goe one link beyond his appointed limitts. If then not hee the master; much less then, any wicked man or woman, who is no better then the slave of that slave. Yet are these miserable miscreants hated by the moste, feared by some, fawned on by others: as if they lyved without the lists or lyberties, of divine power or providence. And on the contrary, the white witches they are admired, applauded, yea well nigh adored (by some of the sottish sorte). And by to many, countenanced, pleaded for and protected.[5] In regard whereof I havc endevoured (according to my poore talent) in this ensuing tract, to discover this mistery of iniquitie; to thend that all Gods people may com to know them, and knowing them, to holde them forever in an abhominable detestation. Beloved its a saying no less ancient then true. *Quj præmonitus, præmunitus: si sapiens sit.*[6] I therefore beseech almighty God of his goodnes, to open the eyes of all that profess his name, that they may be able to discover all the wyles of that wicked one: Hee likewise encourage the harts, and strengthen the hands of all such as are in authority, to cut of these wicked workes from the city of God.

Your servant in the Lord
E. P.

---

[5] See introduction for the context to Poeton's statements about white witches. Complaints about their number and popularity were extremely common among those who wrote about witchcraft in the period. John Cotta, for instance, another physician who published a treatise on the subject, wrote:

> This kinde is not obscure, at this day swarming in the Kingdome, whereof no man can bee ignorant, who lusteth to obserue the vncontrouled libertie and license of open and ordinary resort in all places unto wise-men, and wise-women, so vulgarly termed for their reputed knowledge concerning such diseased persons as are supposed to be bewitched.

The Infallible Trve And Assvred Witch, 69.

[6] Who is forewarned, is forearmed: if he is wise.

[¶3v blank]

[1]

The Winnowing of White Witchcraft.[7]
Handled in forme of a dialouge.[8] *Twixt:*
Dr Dreadnought, a Divine.[9]
Phylomathes, a Physition.[10] *And*
Gregory Groshead, a country Corydon.[11]

Dr:–: Mr *Phylomathes*: I now playnely perceve that you are a man, who is very punctuall in performing, what you promise. You are very welcom unto this place. And I thank you for your paynes, which you bestowed on my selfe, and other your auditors, at our last conference (which wee had at your house) about urines uncertaynties. And now I hope that you will be pleased to afforde us your best notions, for the discovery of white witchcraft.

Phy:–: Reverend Sir: my best abillities rest at your commande. But (in this buisines) I must crave your asistance; because you are better acquainted with the sacred scriptures (by far) then my selfe.

---

[7] Winnowing grain is the process of separating, quite literally, the wheat from the chaff; the term suggests most readily, therefore, separating desirable matter from undesirable. *OED* also records that the term can also be applied to the process of simply getting rid of undesirable material in its own right, however, and this is presumably the sense intended here; there is surely nothing desirable about white witches from which to separate the undesirable material.

[8] For a discussion of the dialogue form, popular among both witchcraft writers and reformers more widely, see introduction.

[9] Dreadnought is not a medical doctor but a Doctor of Divinity, i.e., a clergyman with an advanced level of university education. His surname is an aptronym indicating his fearlessness.

[10] Phylomathes may well be intended to represent Poeton himself. It is a commonly-used name in dialogues (James I had used it for one of the characters in his *Daemonologie*), and derives from the Greek word for a lover of learning ("philomath" in English). It may indicate that this character is subservient to the divine in terms of learning (because the philomath is there to obtain more knowledge by learning from one more educated than he).

[11] "Grosshead" is another aptronym; *OED* records its use in this period as a general term of abuse for a thick-headed person. A corydon is a generic (usually proper) name for a rustic, frequently used in pastoral poetry; see e.g., Milton's "L'Allegro" in John Carey, ed., *Milton: The Complete Shorter Poems* (Harlow: Longman, 2007), l.83.

And those are they, which must be our light and guide, in the way of this discourse.

Dr:–: Sir: you are in the right. And God forbid that I shoulde be backward in this buisines, Ile promise you my best heerin. And loe heere comes one (very opportunely) to speake with mee, as I suppose, who (as I have been informed of late) hath been a greate resorter unto cunning men and woemen: and not onely a greate walker unto Wyzards himself, but also a strong instigator of others, to treade in the same steps, and to pace in the same path. Ile meet him at the doore, and bring him in with mee; And then (if you acorde) weele joyne both our forces together, and in so doing, I trust that (with Gods asistance) wee shall batter the strongest bulwarks that hee hath built up to defend his folly withall. Good morrow neighbour *Gregory*: what good newes with you? Come neare the house I pray you.

Greg:–: Good morrow Mr Dr. An cham glad too zee you well: having zom casion too com this way this morning: I thought good too zatisvye you that aboute *Thurzday* next, I shall ha a good vatt tythe pigg vor yee,[12] an ta may pleaze you too zend vorn than.

Dr:–: Kinde neighbour I thanck you for your paynes. And if your busines be not very important to call you from our company, I shall be glad to have som conference with you, aboute a buisines which more neerly concerns your self then perchance you as yet are aware of.

[2] *Greg*:–: An ta ma pleaze you, Mr Dr my casions bente of any zuch prezent portance, but thats may tarry a while. An that by zo much tha rather, because you tell mee, that there bee zom things, which doo zomwhat nearely conzerne mee: I thong God I know my zelf too bee an onnest man: and all theck while,[13] chill care tha less: let anny boddy ze o mee what a wooll.

Ignorant people, are well conceited of themselves.

Dr:–: Mr *Phylomathes*: seeing that opportunitie offers us, so fitt an occasion, to enter on the pointe, which wee intended to parle aboute, Ile now tell you, what I have been lately certifyed concerning this man: which is, that hee is one who hath often gone unto cunning men and woemen (as the country people use to call them)

[12] i.e., a good fat tithe pig. Tithes were a tax on their parishioners collected by churches, originally paid in kind (hence the offer here of livestock), but by this period tithes could also consist of a money payment. For a discussion of Gregory's dialect, see introduction.

[13] Probably "the eke," using the adverbial form of "eke," meaning "in addition," but slightly twisted by Gregory into an adjective; so roughly meaning "the same while."

to seek help at their hands, when any of his family or frends have been sick: as also that hee is a perswader of others unto the like pernitious practice.

Phy:–: Alas, tis not his case alone: the more is the pitty, and the greater is the iniquitie of theis times. And to tell you the truthe, this land even swarmeth in every countye and corner with white witches: whom thc ignorant people dignifie no les then demy gods, stiling them with the titles of wise or cunning men or woemen.

Greg:–: Whosomever tolde you that I ha gone too witches (zaving your worships reverence) tolde you a starke lye. An vor my parte, I tell yee true, that I hate a witch with all my hart: An I provess that with all my hart, chud bee bounde too carrye a burden of wood zeven myle at my back, to burne won ove um, I love um zo well.[14] Vy uppon um vilthy creturs: tiz ene zin and pitty that the ware nut all ome e burnd. Cha warrant um, I an if all vokes wor o my minde, chud zoone make a hond ome, zo chud.

Dr:–: I pray you neighbour tell mee: who are those that you are so hott against?

Greg:–: Marry zur: the are a zorte a people ene az bad, or worse az the d'vle en zelf. O vy on um vilty creturs, the care nut an the kill bothe man and bease.

Its onely the black witch: that is hated by the common people.

Dr:–: Oh, now I have founde out your meaning. It seems you think that there are no witches besides those who have a hand in doing hurt.

Greg:–: Zur: yee ar in tha right: Ize dee think zo indeed. An too make good my pinnion: I verily beleeve, that noe witch can doo any good, much las the d'vle en zelf.

Dr:–: From your speech it may be collected: that you are conceited, that those wise men and woemen, which you so often have walkt unto: are not witches.

[3] *Greg:*–: I think zo indeed. And vor my parte I never zaw eny harm by um: theyle tawke o God as well as tha best ome all: An I

---

14 Witches in England were hanged, not burned, but this may be Gregory's mistake, rather than Poeton's. Witches were burned in continental Europe and in Scotland, and this seems to have been a part of the popular stereotype in the period, as it is now. The wife of the rustic character in George Gifford's *Dialogve concerning Witches and Witchcraftes* (1593) expresses very similar sentiments, and Gifford knew full well that hanging was the punishment for witchcraft: "If I had but one fagot in the world, I would carry it a myle vpon my shoulders to burne a witch." Gifford, *Dialogve*, D1^{v}. This echo is a possible indication that Poeton had read Gifford's work.

The common people, do much respect white Witches, and are ready to make apologies for them.

ha hurd um ze good prayers meny a time and oft.[15] An vor ought at I zee, a man may speed better at there honns: than if a shud go too won o your vine *vizichians*. An o this cham shure, that the can tell moore of a zick mans state by his water, than won o yeer costly zilken docturs can. Where vore I zee no reazon that won shud bee vounde vaute with vor going too zuch good people: vor the dee pitty a poore boddyes case: I an the wooll doo moore vor vive shillins, than yoer *vizichyans* an pottecarriers wooll doo vor vorty; zo the wooll.[16]

Dr:–: Neighbour *Gregorie*: geve mee leave to goe along with you a littell: and to answere those your secret apollogies which you have made in defence, bothe of your self, and of those your cunning creatures. And whereas (first) you say that you see no harme by them: I doe not much marvayle at your so saying, for (to deale playnely with you) I think that your simplicity is such, that you are not able (in this matter) to discerne twixt good and evill, I think that you are blinde herein.

Greg:–: Who: I blinde? zaving your worships revarence. I dare boldly zay, that I can zee az well az your zelfe, I thonk God.

Dr:–: Mistake mee not: for I no way intend the bodily or outward sight: but the inwward and spirituall illumination of the minde. For were you enlightned with grace from above: you woulde not so magnifie those pestilent kinde of people as you doe: and that because they often name God and Christ, you think them to be goode people. But I pray you to tell mee, hath not the devill himself often used as good wordes as possibly they can? And yet notwithstanding, you cannot but acknowledg that hee is a devill still. And to make good what I say. I pray you dilligently to observe the deportment of the devill towards our blessed Saviour, in the dayes of

[15] The use of prayers and other religious language by white witches was common, given that the vast majority of magical rituals and charms had their source in the Bible, religious ceremonies, and other less orthodox Christian imagery. Both scholarly and popular magic were steeped in the language of prayer and scripture. See Davies, *Popular Magic*; Wilson, *The Magical Universe*; Thomas, *Religion and the Decline of Magic*; Bardell, "Beyond Pendle" in Poole, ed., *The Lancashire Witches*, and any of the sources cited elsewhere in this volume on ritual magic or charms.

[16] Complaints about the expense of physicians were fairly typical during the period: they were genuinely expensive. Nicholas Culpeper, for example (an unlicensed physician), comments on "the medicines of the College of Physicians that are so dear and scarce to finde." Nicholas Culpeper, *The English Physician* (London: William Bentley, 1652), 10.

his flesh: and if you be not willfully obstinate, you will soone assent unto this truthe. Wherefore to make it the more playnely to appeare unto you; Ile instance in som particulars, which you shall see to be sett downe, in sacred writt.

The often using of the name of God: no certayne note of a sounde hart.

Beholde heere what is recorded by St *Mark ch.* 1. *ver.* 24. the latter parte of the verse. *Sathans* wordes (unto our Saviour) are theis: *I know thee who thou art, the holy one of God.* Againe *Mark* 5. 7. *Jesus thou sonn of the moste high God.* Againe see heere *Luke* 8. 28. (mark the wordes) *When he saw Jesus, he cryed out, and fell downe before him, and with a loude voyce sayd, what have I to doe with thee, Jesus, thou sonn of the moste high God? I beseech thee torment mee not.* Loe heere you see that the devill confesseth Jesus, falls downe before him, yea **[4]** earnestly beseecheth him not to torment him. Consider likewise the devills demeanour towards the disciples of our blessed saviour. Loe heere *Acts* 16. 17. the devill confesseth St Paule and his companions: *To be the servants of the moste high God: which shew unto us the way of salvation &c.* Now if the devill thus freely, and frequently confess Christ; and made request unto him with such earnest observations, shall wee need to doubt, that hee will deny his disciples, to imitate his actions. Know oh know for an infallible truthe, that many Hypocrites and Helhoundes, make as fayre a shew of sanctitie, as the best of Gods servants can doe, yet shall they not be saved thereby. *For it is not every one that sayth Lord Lord, that shall enter into the kingdome of heaven*: its onely those, *who doe the will of God which is in heaven. Matthew* 7. 21. Its fayth in the hart & the fruites thereof in the life which pleaseth God. And whereas you affirme, that they often say good prayers: I much distrust your judgment in matter of prayer: I greately feare, (that your simplicitie is such) that you know not what prayer is.

The common people, are for the moste part ignorant; and know not what prayer is.

Greg:–: Cham zorry master doctor, that you shud ha zuch a conzete o mee: I tell ee truely (I thong God vort) I dee ze my prayers ery morning, whan I wash my vace an honns, An zo agen at night whan cham abed: An cham shure that the bee good prayers too, vor the bee zuch az you your zelf dee uze too ze in tha church. An if theise bee nut good prayers, than lord ha marcy uppons all.

Dr:–: Without some speciall grace from above, I plainly perceve, that it will prove a very tedious task, to informe and reforme you, (and such as you are) for as far as I can conjecture, ignorance and obstinacye, are conjoyned in you. But pray tell mee what are those prayers, which your wise woemen use to say?

Greg:–: Why zur: the bee zuch as I uze too ze my zelf.

Dr:–: And what are those I pray you?

Greg:–: Cha tolde ee wonce a reddy: an cham nut aveard too tell you what the bee: vor an ee wooll needs know. Tiz *Our Vather* &c. An *I beleeve in God* &c. *Hayle Mary* vull a grace &c.[17] An zum wother zuch leek good prayers, which ha no hurt in um, cham zure a that, zo cham.

Dr:–: Alas poore man I much pitty your absurd ignorance: But God assisting mee, I will doe the best that I can to draw you from out of this **[5]** dangerous snare of the devill, in the which you are sorely intangled, although you discerne it not: I know that you have often heard it, though you little heeded it. Wherefore I will now (once agayne) shew you that which I require you to take speciall notice of. See heere what St Paule hath sett downe in his second epistle to the Corinthians *ch.* 11. *ver.* 14. *For Sathan is transformed*

[17] The paternoster, Creed, and Ave Maria. While the former two were still in use in English Protestant services, the latter of these three is explicitly Catholic. This is presumably the reason for the divine's reaction, but it may also be a reaction to the use of prayers in an inappropriate situation. In this instance Gregory's excuse seems to be merely ignorance—though this was not considered a valid excuse in such matters (see 35)—but Catholic prayers and rituals were often associated with diabolism in their own right. Bernard, for example, in a list of those most likely to become witches, includes:

> Those that bee superstitious and idolatrous, as all Papists be. That of these very many the Diuell works vpon to make Witches, is not to be doubted: for Sorcery is the practice of that Whore, the Romish Synagogue, Reuel. 18. 23. Secondly, it is found true, that healing Witches doe vse many of their superstitious Ceremonies, Lip-prayers, Aue-Maries, Creeds, and Pater-nosters by set numbers. Thirdly, when Poperie beare sway heere, then Diuels and Spirits often appeared, and at that time were many more Witches then now.

Bernard, *A Gvide To Grand-Ivry Men*, 99–100.

The "*Pater noster, Ave, and Credo*" are to be used, to give a practical example, in a ritual to bind the spirit of a dead person to one's service, cited by Reginald Scot in his *Discouerie of witchcraft* (1584), bk. 15, chap. 17. Scot's book was a compendium of rituals and charms, based on extensive research with manuscript grimoires and other magical texts; Scot, however, published them in order that their self-evident absurdity would be apparent (Scot was extremely sceptical about the powers of witches, ascribing all supposedly supernatural occurrences either to Providence or trickery). By the 1630s the association of Catholicism with diabolism was bound up in the Calvinist attack on the Arminian ascendancy, led by Archbishop Laud, which saw a greater focus on ritual and ceremony in church practices, and which, its opponents argued, was but a hair's breadth from papistry. Poeton, a Calvinist, may have this context in mind here.

into an angell of light. And this I know, that Sathan will not onely allow, but often instigate his servants unto a shew of sanctitie.

Phy:–: I can witnes the same uppon myne owne knowledge.

Dr:–: Neighbour *Gregory*, what say you to this? doe you think that your wise woemen may be deceived (themselves) by Sathan in taking him to be an Angell of light: and so delude you, and such as you are?

Greg:–: Think nut: I dee think the bee good vokes, zo I doe.

Dr:–: Well I trust that (er many dayes pass over) I shall bring you into another minde. But to pass this; Ile now touche uppon another pointe of your apologie. I remember that you sayde that one mought speed better at their hands, then at the hands of a fine *Physition* which you did instance in ii perticulars. Viz. 1. In that they are better skild in the judgment of urines. 2. That it is far cheaper to goe unto them. Now neighbour, I pray you tell mee, how such kinde of people (as generally such are) who have very littell learning; shoulde be able to discerne more by an urine, then wise, learned, and judicious *Physitions* can doe?

Whence shoulde such have this skill?

Greg:–: Why: I think that tiz a gift that God ha ginn um, too doo poore vokes good withall. Vor an the had nut a gift vrom God, the coude nere know zo much az the doo know; nor zure, the wood nere doo zo much good az the doo.

The sottish conceit of many countrey people, who thinke that white witches are illumined from above.

Dr:–: Neighbour *Gregory*: you think that they have their skill as a gift geven unto them by God: But in this you speake without any sacred sence. For God worketh not now in theis dayes by miracle but by meanes; for miracles have long since seiced:[18] and when that it pleased almighty God to bestow the gift of miracles uppon his church; those on whom hee bestowed the same, were ever such, as were his blessed instruments to establish his law; or to propogate his gospell. But **[6]** blessed be God, the gospell hath long since been established with us, and there is no need of miracles to mayntaine

[18] The cessation of miracles was a widely-held Protestant viewpoint, though it was not quite as simple as absolute cessation, as Alexandra Walsham has shown in *Providence in Early Modern England* (Oxford: Oxford University Press, 1999), 226–32. It was an argument often made in the context of attacks on Catholicism and superstition. Briefly, the argument ran thus: that since the miracles of Christ and the Apostles (those of the latter effected not via their own power but by God working through them) were enough to confirm the truth of the scriptures, there was no longer any requirement for further miracles, and religion should be based on faith in the Gospel alone. For an example of this argument, see James I, *Daemonologie*, 66.

it: God worketh now by ordinary meanes: In regarde whereof it is meet, that a *Physition* be furnished with a compotent measure of knowledg in the nature of Simples,[19] (yea its fitt that hee well know the simples themselves, for otherwise, the common countrye people will often mistake; and that not without greate perrill unto the patient). Its also necessary, that hee be furnished with the motions of such severall sicknesses, as are incident unto the body of man: and that they be likewise well verst in the sundry Symptomes, signes, and marks of each severall maladye; which to attayne, requires long and dilligent studye, with manifolde experience, conjoyned with a carefull observation of all passages and opperations.

Now theis things considered, whence (think you) shoulde these illiterate Ideots, get that profuseness of knowledg: which you (and such as you are) so much dignifie and extoll? How can they attayne to that height of excellency in the Uromantike art; as that they shoulde be able uppon the sole sight of a carryed urine, to discover each particuler that a poore patient is either pincht or plagued withall? Can this be done without some complication with Sathan? What think you now of this matter neighbour *Gregory*?

Greg:–: Think ote, what shud I think ote? I think az I thought avore; I an cham verely purzwaded, zo cham, that tiz God that dee help um: ze what ee wooll. An vor my parte chill nere ze wotherwize than cha vounde (nor no boddyes plesur) vor I nere zaw eny harme they did: no nor, I nere hurd eny harme they zed. I think that tiz a zin to beelye tha d'vle. I can zee no reazon why I shud be perzwaded too think ill o zuch good vokes az the bee. I An I know what I know well enough, zo I doo.

Dr:–: And what is that which you know so well? I pray you let mee be so much beholding unto you, as to know it also.

Greg:–: Why master doctur, too tell ee true, az I may zay too you; cha zeen menny a good man an woman too, I an that of **[7]** no small steem in tha world: I, an zuch, az think themzelves az wize az your worship that goe too um az well az I. An if twere zuch a vawte, az you ze tiz: I think that zuch wize vokes wood nere goe too um. An there bee nut a vew zuch nother, I may tell you.

The example of great ones, is a greate encouragement, to the common people to doe evill.

Dr:–: Neighbour, Neighbour: and I must needs tell you, that either you know not, or els you forget (if you doe not contemne) the commandement of the Almighty: which is this. *Thou shalt not follow a multitude to doe evill. Exodus ch.* 23. *ver.* 2.

[19] Medicinal plants or herbs.

Greg:–: Vor all at you ha zed: I donte think that tiz eny vawte too goe too those good vokes. An az I zed avore, I zee that ery dey az wise vokes az moste bee, doe bothe goe too um: I, and zend vor um whom too ther houzen, I, an wooll take thur device avore that the wooll take your zilken docturs pinnion. An ee cante make mee beeleeve that zuch wise vokes wood goe too um, an if the ware witches, az you wood vayne parzwade mee too think. An I zeate agenn that vor my parte I nere zaw no zuch thing by um: nother doe I think that tiz eny zinn too goe too um: zea what you wooll.

The common sorte, holde it no sinn to goe to witches.

Dr:–: Alas poore man, I much pitty your case: for I now playnlie perceve that ignorance and obstinacy, is the groundeworke of your building: the wills and workes of men, are the walls and windows thereof, and the covering is nothing els but your owne self conceite. And you have planchered it,[20] with the practices of unregenerate persons; which you prefer before the precepts of the most high and most holy God. Whence it cometh to pass that God in justice hath suffered Sathan so to besott you, that you see it not (as yet) to bee any sinn.

Greg:–: Too tell ee true (without eny simulation) I donte think that tiz a zinn, too goe too um vor helpe.

Dr:–: I confess (but alas the more is the pitty) that you are not the first that hath erred in this kinde. For I have just cause to feare, that many thowsand soules have perished, by walking in theis wayes of wickednes. Alas this error is ancient, and many princes **[8]** and Potentates, have been seduced by Sathan: And that not onely some heathen, but also sundry such as have made an outward profession of true religion, and have lyved within the pale of the holy church of God. And for your better instruction I will shew you sundry such as I finde to be registred and recorded in sacred writt. Wherefore first to begin with the first that I finde to be sett downe since the fall of our first parents, who was *Pharaoh* king of Egipt: who when God sent *Moses* unto him to require or charge him (in the name of the Lord) to lett Israell departe from out his land and service. The king (as may be gathered from the text) uppon the hearing of this Embassie, required a miracle, at the hands of the Ambassadors. Whereuppon, *Aaron* (as the Lord had foredirect) cast downe his rod before *Pharaoh and it became a serpent*. As heere you may see sett downe *Exodus* 7. 10. Whereuppon *Pharaoh* called for the wise men and the sorcerers: who by their enchantments did the like as *Aaron* had done: for they cast downe every man his rod

Princes and Potentates, have been seduced by Sathan.

20 Covered or floored with wooden planks (here used figuratively).

and they became *serpents*: but *Aarons* rod swallowed up their rodds. *ver.* 11. *et* 12. Loe heer (neighbour *Gregory*) you see a mighty monarch consulting with theis witches. And agayne you likewise see, that by the power of *Sathan*, those witches counterfeited Gods true miracle. Againe, beholde heere ver. 22. those Magicians (in shew) turned the waters into blood. Again *ch.* 8 *ver.* 7. those Magicians brought up froggs uppon the the land of Egipt. And again *ver.* 18. brought Lyce by their enchantments. Loe heer good neighbour you may see the power and policy of *Sathan* in theis witches, his instruments. But to proceed: you may reade *Numbers* 22. 5. &c. of *Balaam* the sonn of *Beor*: for whom *Balak* king of *Moab* sent the elders of his people. And againe. *ver.* 15. hee sent yet againe Princes moe and more honourable then the former. And *ver.* 36. *Balak* the king went to meet him in person: and ascribes unto *Balaam* the power of blessing and cursing. Loe heer a very greate deale of honour. 1. done by this king: unto this wicked wretch: who (as *St Peter* sayth) *loved the wages of unrighteousness*. 2. *Peter* 2. 15. This was that *Balaam who taught Balak, to lay a stumbling block before the* **[9]** *children of Israell. Revelations* 2. 14. In sum hee was a false prophet yea a very white witch. Againe in the first book of *Samuell ch.* 28. *ver.* 3. wee may reade of such as had familiar spiritts, and of wizards. Yea even in the bosome of the church of God. And doubtles theis were not without their clyents, yea even of such as made an outward profession of Gods pure worship and service. And if wee looke unto *ver.* 7. wee shall finde that King Saul enquired for a woman who had a familiar spirit. And in *ver.* 8. you may reade, how that hee disguised himself and went to Endor unto a *witch* and consulted with her. Againe in the second book of Kings *ch.* 21. *ver.* 6. you may reade of *Manasseh king of Iudah, who was an observer of times, a user of enchantments: and a dealer with familiar spirits, and with wizards.* Agayne, in the second chapter of the holy prophet *Daniell* at *ver.* 10. you may reade of *Magicians; Astrologers: and Caldeans*, alowed of, if not maintayned by; King *Nebuchadnezzar* that greate king of *Babylon*: As also his sending for them: his consulting with them. Againe in the fift chapter of *Daniell* at *ver.* 7 &c. you may read of *Belshazzar* the king of *Babylon*: who (having seen the handwriting uppon the wall) *cryed aloude to bring in the Astrologers, the Caldeans, and the Soothsayers to reade the writing* &c. Agayne you may reade in the *Acts* of the holy *Apostles. ch.* 8. *ver.* 9. &c. of *Simon Magus the sorcerer who bewitched the people of Samaria in such sorte that they all gave heed unto him from the leaste unto the greatest, accounting him to be the greate power of God.* Agayne *ch.* 13. *ver.* 6. &c. you may reade of one *Barjesus, or Elymas a sorcerer, who was in greate esteem*

Unregenerate men are ready to deifie the devils disciples.

with Sergius Paulus the deputie of Paphos. Againe *ch*. 16. et *ver*. 16. &c. you may read of a certayne damosell, *who was possessed with a spiritt of divination, by which much gaynes came to her masters*. Now in that it is sayde that much gaine came unto her masters: It must then follow by necessary consequence, that there was greate resorte unto her, high esteem of her. So as now (from all theis instances) I may safely conclude that it is not a thing either new or strange, for greate persons to runn a whoring after witches: neither is it any marvayle unto mee **[10]** that a man of your meane capacitie shoulde be seduced, and so led aside by theis lying and bewitching vanities. For you see that many princes, potentates, and peeres, with much people, of all suites and sortes, have been (from tyme to tyme) seduced, beguiled, and deceved, by that enemy unto (and decever of) mankinde, I meane that olde Serpent the devill *who goeth aboute continually like a roaring lyon, seeking whom hee may devoure*. 1. *Peter* 5. 8. Wherefore I admonish and advise you (my good neighbour, whose soule is deare unto Christ, as having cost him the price of his moste precious blood. And it is (and ought to be) much respected of mee, who am your *Pastor*, and am bounde (in that respect) to have a speciall care of your soule, knowing that I must geve an accounte unto God for the same). Oh that you woulde seriously consider of theis thinges, and lay them unto hart, and that you may so doe, I pray to God that hee will (in mercy) vouchsafe so to open the eyes of your understanding, that you may be able to trye theis spirits whether they be of God or no, according as you are therto exhorted by that holy and blessed *Apostle* and *Evangelist* St *John*, in his first *Epistle ch*. 4. *ver*. 1. Oh good neighbour: be not carryed away (any longer) with the common cursed conceites of vayne and unregenerate people, whose wisdome is but earthly, sensuall, and devillish. As St *James* speaketh, in the third chapter of his Epistle *ver*. 15. And know this, that whosoever they bee that run unto theis kinde of people, (putting their confidence in them) doe make themselves thereby, an abomination unto the Lord. Tell mee, what say you to these thinges?

Pastors ought to have care of the soules of such as are committed to their charge.

Greg:–: *Why zur*: *Ize* must needes convess that I nere hurd zo much avore in all my life: But it vor all that you ha zed: I can scace beeleeve, that theis wise vokes shud bee zo bad az you wood zeem too make um: vor too tell ee true zur, cha knowne menny zuch in my dese, anz nere zee no hurt by um. An theres now a good woman that lives nut vur vro *Gnikrad*:[21] chave e bee with hur menny a time

[21] Read in reverse this is Darking, i.e., Dorking, in Surrey, a market town around twenty-five miles north-east of Petworth. In *The Vrinall*

an oft, an it, I nere zee no hurt by her; shees a very good boddy, chill ze that vor er, I an won that duz a greate deale a good too menny poore vokes, zo shee duth. Can tha d'vle doo enny good zur?

The devill cannot doe any thing thats truely good.

[11] *Dr*:–: No, certainly the devill cannot doe any thing thats truely good:[22] the reason whereof is, because hee is wholely evill. The which notwithstanding (by the Allmighties permission) hee is able *to transforme himself into the likeness of an angell of light*. 2. *Corinthians* 11. 4. And hee is so subtill a *serpent* that (if it were possible) hees able to seduce the very elect, as our saviour sayde. *Mark* 13. 22. So that (for my parte) I am verely perswaded: that (God permitting) the devill can direct and apply, the spirits and vertues, either of vegitables or mineralls, unto the health and recovery of the bodyes, either of man or beast. And I no less beleeve, but that the devil will be very industrious to be an instrument of bodily health, either unto man or beaste, if in the interim; hee can (by any sleight or stratagem) wreake, hurt, or wounde the soule.

The devill will willingly help the body, if that thereby hee may hurt the soul.

Greg:–: Vor my parte, tho cha but a littell lurning, it I deny tha d'vle an alls works. An I thong God, cha lurnd too bless my zelf from tha d'vle, ery morning zoa zoone az cham up: In tha name o the vather: an o the zunn: an o tha holy *ghost*; amen.

Dr:–: Alas poore man, I profess that I am right sorry for the state of your poore soule, I did not think that there had been so much absurditie and ignorance in you. I thought to have taken some other time to have talkt with you, but seeing that in delay, often lyeth danger, and that its best taking Time by the foretop, Ile entreate *Mr Phylomathes* to asist mee with his best advice, for the cure of this miserable maladie.

Phy:–: *Reverend Sir*: this mans sicknes is in his soule; and the phisick which hee needeth is spirituall, which you (Mr Dr) are better able (by far) than my self to administer unto him. The which notwithstanding my poore mite rests at your commande.

---

crackt in the carriage Poeton mentions "my olde Dame of Darking," presumably a local cunning woman or healer, and it is no doubt the same person he refers to here. He goes on to describe her (with extreme sarcasm) as "the very Diamond of Darking, the extract of art, the quintessence of cunning . . . the most pragmaticall pissprophetes. that these southern parts possesses." Sloane MS 1954, §3, 19, 30.

[22] The secondary annotator (see introduction) adds an important rider to Poeton's marginal note here: "nor any thing w^th^out gods permiss[i]on."

Dr:–: Kinde Sir: I thanck you for your courtesie. But neighbour *Gregory*, I pray you tell mee whether you think your self in any faulte, in your often walking unto those wise folkes?

The common sorte think it to be no sinn to goe unto white witches.

Greg:–: No shure I donte thinke that chwaz in enny vawte in going to zeek vor help, and health vrom zuch az can doo won good.

[12] *Dr:–*: It seems that you are perswaded that those people which you have so often gone unto, are noe witches.

Greg:–: I think that theres noo boddy that dare ze the ar witches. An vor my parte, I must needs zay that I nere zaw no hurt in um, zo I did nut; An why shud I ze otherwise than I ha vounde by um; chill nere zeat while I leeve, zo I wonte.

Dr:–: But of this I am sure that you cannot be ignorant, that they are without learning; And that what they doe cannot then be done by lawfull meanes, hath been already proved unto you. Wherefore I say that unles you can shew us better reasons for your going unto them then hitherto you have done: you have very much offended Almightie God therein.

Greg:–: I donte think zo, nut I.

Dr:–: I require you to mark dilligently whats heer written in holy Scripture. See heer. *Leviticus* 19. 31. *Regard not them that have familiar spirits: neither seek after wizards to be defiled by them.* See heer agayne. *Leviticus* 20. 6. *And the soule that runneth after such as have familiar spirits, and after wizards, to goe a whoring after them: I will even set my face against that soule, and will cut him of from among his people.* What think you now neighbour *Gregory*?

Greg:–: I think that you ha too much lurning vor mee: I cante holde argation[23] wee, nut I.

Dr:–: I see that your wise enough to wrong your self and your owne poore soule. But answere mee directly. Doth God forbid going to such people or not?

Greg:–: Yes I think a doo vorbid going too witches and wizards. But I thong God I nere went too enny zuch, that I know on.

Dr:–: I think that you cannot deny but that you have been often with the woman of *Guikrad*: And with her of *Drofrik*. And with her of *Mahpots*. And with the man at *Mahkaht* (when hee was lyving).[24] And you likewise perswaded others to goe unto them.

---

[23] Apparently a nonce-word, or perhaps a colloquialism. Its meaning is clear from context: argument, debate, etc.

[24] More reversed place-names. Drofrik (spelt Drofdrik later on) is Kirdford, a West Sussex village around four miles northeast of Petworth, mentioned later in the text. The others are Stopham and Thakeham, villages around four miles southeast and ten miles east of Petworth, respec-

Greg:–: I donte deny but that cha gon too um all: An cha zent zum too um too. But that I ze iz this, I donte think that the wore enny witches.

[13] *Dr*:–: I confess that it is a very difficult matter (point blank) to prove any one to be a witch, unless it be uppon confession of the delinquent, which is very rare. But there are certayne probable presumptions, whereby through their practice it may be collected that such people as those are, cannot attayne unto such extraordinary science, without som extraordinary helps. And in this I woulde have you to tell mee but this one thing: that is, how your wise woemen shoulde be able, uppon the meere inspection of an urine, (which hath been brought unto them many myles, whose contents have been broken, and confused) that they shoulde (I say) be able to tell, any greef that a sick person is infested withall. And whence they shoulde have that exquisitenes of art, as to prescribe or geve, fitting, proper, and convenient medicines, for the cure of any disease. And that in this regarde, that such silly woemen are unlearned, and ignorant, of the knowledge of the first rudiments or principles of that honourable art. By what meanes think you, that they shoulde have such greate skill?

This is a sure signe of a white witch.

Greg:–: Why, I can ze no more than cha zed a reddy. Zure, I think tiz a gift God han geen um: I ca-nte ze how it shud bee wotherwize.

Dr:–: This triviall tenet of yours, hath already, sufficiently been answered. And it hath been playnly proved unto you, that God worketh now (in theis times) by meanes, and not by miracle.

The good opinion that the common people have of those wise woemen, on what it is grounded.

Greg:–: Why zur: I donte ze that the doo worke by miracle, cham shure that the uze meanes, I, an that good meanes too: An too proove that I ze too bee true, vor myne none part chill zee thuz much vor um, that cha had good oyntments, an good zeercloathes[25] vrom um: An cha had good powders, an holsom earbs: I, an (I may tell you) az good drenches[26] vor won thats zick, az enny boddy can dezire. An vor ought that I can zee, thele geeve az good destructions how too order ery thing az tha best doctor ome all.

tively. Perhaps the names are disguised to prevent Poeton's readers from attempting to visit the white witches? The cunning woman at Kirdford is mentioned later in the treatise as Gammer Tnuh (i.e., Hunt). I am grateful to Luap Nniuq for assistance with the place-names.

25 Cerecloths, a type of plaster applied to bruises, aches, sprains, and similar injuries. With thanks to Jennifer Evans.

26 Medicinal draughts or potions.

An bente thease good meanes think you, I marle much what you wood ha moore?

Dr:–: Now you think that you have built a strong bulwark indeed, for their defence: But I will trye whether it will abyde the battery or not. I doubt not, but that reason will rase it even unto the very foundation. What say you to this argument? Those who want learning and knowledg in the rules of Art, and yet (ordinarily as you affirme) effect **[14]** cures, must needs have som extraordinary help: But theis kind of people want learning, and knowledg in the rules of art (and yet as you affirme effect cures). Therefore theis people, must needs have some extraordinary help.

Greg:–: Why zur: zo I think the ha: vor the bee wise voke I can tell ee.

Dr:–: Alas neighbour: this wisdome that you attribute unto them, is not from above: But it is (as formerly hath been shewed unto you) sensuall, worldly, and devilish. And whereas you object that they use meanes, as oyntments &c. Theis are nothing els but Sathanicall sleights to vizor their witchcraft withall. And its well knowne, that they have very few medicines, against all those manifolde maladies, which the bodyes of men are subject unto. But now lett mee ask you another question: did you never heare any of them profess themselves able to help such as were bewitched?

A strong reason to perswade the common people, to resorte unto white witches.

Greg:–: Yes that I ha: An (I tell ee true) I like um nere tha worse vor that. Vor cha knowne zum my zelf, that ha lost there cattell strangely, and nere cud gett enny help vort, till zuch time az the went too zum o theis good vokes, and zunce that: there cattell ha dun very well. An won thing I commend um vor: that is, the bee willing too tell won what shall doome good: An theres won trick above the rest, that I trust God wooll bless um vor: vor ta dun tha cuntry abominable good. An beecause that (I trust) ee bee my vrends, chill tell ee what tiz. I can tell ee that within these vorty yeares, cha known (my zelf) menny groundes, which ha bee haunted by d'vles (az I think) that looke what ever cattell were put intoo um: wor shure too dy vort. Till zuch time az these good vokes tought how too help it. An too make short ote, twaz no wother than this. The bid um to make a vayre cross uppon ery tree, that stood in tha hedges quite rounde aboute tha veilde, an zo a good menny ha dun: An uppon my knowledg the that did zo, nere lost enny o ther cattell zunce, for tiz zartayne that that *Puxxe* hath no power too com into enny grounde whare tha trees bee zo crost.[27] Now chud

[27] A puck, or puckrel, is a type of mischievous spirit. Shakespeare's Robin Goodfellow in *A Midsummer Night's Dream* (written c. 1595, first

vayne zee, zum o your vine *vizichians*, doo tha cuntry zo much good in enny won thing.

A History.

Phy:–: *Worthy Sir*: this mans speech brings a matter to my remembrance, which (with your leave) Ile now declare unto you. There was (well neare forty yeares since) a certayne professed Artist,[28] (with whom I had familiar acquaintance, as being my countryman) who then dwelt in the *Priory* house of *Stokeclare* in *Suffolk.*[29] This gentillman was a master of Arts, and a *Licenciate* bothe in *Physick and chyrurgerie.*[30] Hee likewise **[15]** profest (though not publikely) the cure of *Witchcraft*. Yea and closely underhand, the revealing of secrets concerning things stolln. *Greate* resorte there was unto him: And much help the country aboute him, obtayned by him, in cheef concerning man or beaste which were bewitched. Now after some iii or iiii yeares had confirmd our first auquayntance; wee hapned (aboute the spring time of the yeare) to meet together not far from London. And as wee walked together viewing the groundes, bancks, and hedges, hee sodaynely stopt, and somwhatt passionately laught. I entreating a reason of his soddayne myrth: hee shewed mee a plant, not long before put forth, and asked of mee if I knew it? I answered yes. Then hee further demanded of mee, if I did not remember a certayne plott of grounde which lay between his house at *Clare* and the castell ditch, wherein grew som plenty of that plant.[31] I answered him that I did remember it. Then

printed 1600) is of course the most famous example; Ben Jonson's unfinished play *The Sad Shepherd* (first printed in the second edition of his *Workes*, 1641) also features a character called Puck-hairy. The rustic speaker in Gifford's *Dialogve* refers to a witch said to have "three or foure imps, some call them puckrels," B1ʳ. Thomas Heywood's *Hierarchie of the blessed Angells* (London: Adam Islip, 1635) briefly discusses "Pugs and Hob-goblins," 574.

[28] In this context, a person skilled in the magical or occult arts. Poeton will return to this term later in the work.

[29] Stoke-by-Clare, a small village in the southwest corner of Suffolk, in the valley of the river Stour. This passage perhaps indicates that Poeton lived in Suffolk at some point or at least had spent some time there.

[30] This indicates that the man in question was both university-educated and a legally respectable physician who also performed the office of surgeon. He is of similar status to Poeton himself; while Poeton does not appear to have attended university, he describes himself as "Licentiate in Physick and Chyrurgery" in Bonham, *The Chyrvrgians Closet*, a3ʳ. See introduction.

[31] Clare is a southwest Suffolk town on the banks of the Stour, around two miles east of Stoke-by-Clare.

hee tolde mee that (many times) hee had gott moneys thereby. I askt him how? Why quoth hee when people came unto mee, for their cattell when they were bewitched (as they thought) I then commonly went unto that plott of grounde, and there gatherd such hearbes as first came to hand, whereof there was the greatest plenty of that plant; and so delyverd them, to such as came, together with some directions for their use, and so (taking their moneys) dismisst them. I then entreated him truely to tell mee, whether there were any plants endowed with such vertue as to cure witchcraft. Hee ingeniously confest the contrarye; and tolde mee in playne termes; that hee never regarded what hee gave them, but onely relyed uppon certayne rules of his art: The which were (as I afterwards fisht from him) certayne charmes, and spells, (which hee called prayers) and other such like devillish dotages. But som outward meanes hee ever used, to none other end then to palliate his pernitious practises. And theis things doe I speake uppon my owne knowledg.

Dr:–: Neighbour *Gregory*: what say you of this story: doe you think it to be true or not?

[16] *Greg*:–: Ta ma bee true vor ought at I know.

Dr:–: I know not any reason that may move you to make any doubte thereof. Wherefore I playnely pronounce unto you, that you have sinned against God, in going unto witches.

Greg:–: I do-nte think that the be witches: vor cham shure o that, that cha hurd um speake az much agenst witches az enny boddy can, and that nut wonce or twyce, but menny a time an oft. I, and zom time thele nut stick too tell there names too, too a vrend or zo: shure the bee good vokes, I ze still.

Dr:–: Loe now you have sayde enough: for it is apparant from that which you have spoken, that they can bee no better then white witches: els how shoulde they com to know, who be black or hurting witches, if the devill did not geve them information thereof?

Greg:–: I must ene convess, that you ha sposde me: But it vor all that: tho I bee but a zimple Scholler, it I thong God, I can remember zum what o that, chave e hurd red in tha church, zoas can.

Dr:–: And what is that which you remember?

An Objection

Greg:–: Marry zur: chill tell ee what: (An I dee think that ee wooll bee of another minde whan you heear what tiz) did nut our zaviour Christ zay, that Zatans kingdome iz nut devided agenst en zelf: vor if a shud (az hee did zay) a coude nut stand?[32] What zay too this Master doctor?

---

32 Gregory refers to Matthew 12:26.

Dr:–: I confess as much, But what doe you infer uppon it?

Greg:–: Inveer uppont, marry chill tell ee whats dee inverr uppont. If these good vokes wor witches, az you wood zeem to make um, than the wood nere speak zo much agenst witches az the doo: noe nor the wood nere tell there vrends whoo hurt um: vor in zo dooing (in my zimple understanding) Zatans kingdome shud bee devided: which an if it wonce cum too that pass, than hiz kingdom cannut stand. Wooll ee make mee beleeve that Zatan iz zuch a voole, az that a wooll doo enny thing to overthrow hiz owne kingdome?

Reasons to strengthen the objection.

Answere, by similitude.

Dr:–: You have now spoken somwhat learnedly indeed. And I see that you have witt enough to couzin your self and wrong your owne soule. You conceite that one witches maligning of another, and their discovering **[17]** of one another, is such a division that Sathans kingdome will thereby be overthrowne. But heerin you are much mistaken, as by a fitt and familiar similitude I shall soone make it apparant unto you.

Greg:–: An if I bee zo much mistaken, az you make wize that I am: pray show mee wharein, an how; An than chill ze zo too.

Dr:–: Neighbour: you know well enough, that in every earthly kingdome, there is a king: there are princes: peeres: privy counsellors: subordinate magistrates: and common people.

Greg:–: All this I know: An what of all this I pray?

Dr:–: You know likewise that in such a kingdom, many of the common sorte of people doe often fall out among themselves, vex one another by suites in law: traduce and slander one another: yea somtimes strike, wounde, kill one another: yet nevertheles the state stands still in securitie, so long as the king, princes, peeres, &c. accorde and agree well among themselves.

Greg:–: Ee ze well an wizely: But whats all this too tha d'vles kingdome?

Dr:–: I apply the similitude thus: There is in the kingdome of the devill, a principall head or king, who in the sacred scripture is called *Baalzebub*, or *Beelzebub*, as wee see him so stiled *Luke* 11. 15. Under whom there are other wicked spirits, subordinate bothe in place and power unto that their king or head. And theis are stiled, by the holy apostle St *Paule Ephesians* 6. 12. *principalities*; *powers*; rulers of the darknes of this worlde; spirituall wicknesses in high places:[33] theis have their severall circuits, regions, and precints:

[33] The *OED* records usages of "wickness," but in the fourteenth century only; this is probably an error for "wickedness," as in the 1611 translation.

under theis there are common subjects: to witt all the wicked of the earth, even all the children of disobedience, in whose harts Sathan ruleth, as their cheeftayne or soveraygne, and St *Paule* testifyeth *Ephesians* 2. 2. Now theis may: yea and often they do differ among themselves; accusing; calumniating, and persecuting one another, and that with most cruell eagernes, envy, mallyce, and all possible violence that can bee devised: And yet all this, no way to the detriment, but rather to the greater advancement, of Sathans Scepter, and the more spatious and ample enlargement, of his kingdom. Lett mee ask you one thing, did you ever heare or reade that the devills did differ among themselves or dissent one from another: but that they holde themselves still in a moste **[18]** close combination: subtilly conspiring, and sedulously labouring, to worke mans destruction: And now neighbour tell mee, whether you did not much mistake your self in this matter, when you tooke it to be a hurt unto the devills kingdom that one witch shoulde detect another.

Greg:–: Mee thinks chwaz mistaken in tha matter indeed. Too zee; wee ingrant cuntry vokes may think our zelves wizer (menny times) than wee bee indeed. Ile tell ee Mr doctor, I did verrily think that chad e sposde ee. But too tell ee true; that, that ee ha now e zed (I may ze too you), ha cast a shroade quawme over my stummak. I ca-nte tell well what too ze toot. But an chwere shure indeed, that theis wize vokes dud deale wee tha d'vle: chud zee um in a quagmoyre avore zuch time az chud goo too um agen. An now (vor this trick) chill tell ee true. I wonce went, (an nere but wonce thats can remember) untoo my gammer *Tnuh* of *Drofdrik*;[34] an too convess playnely too ee, shee made mee a moaste agast, vor tha pestance[35] woman did whisper and mutter zum things too hur zelf. I ca-nte tell what twaz, nut I. Too tell ee true chad zum spission o tha matter; vor I did nut like hur dooings very well, zo I did nut; An vor that trick I nere came there agen.

Dr:–: It seems then that you doe not reckon your gammer *Tnuh*, in the number of your good vokes: But what think you of all the rest, that you have gone too?

[34] Drofdrik is Kirdford (see above, note 24). In *The Vrinall crackt in the carriage*, alongside the "Dame of Darking," Poeton mentions "mother Hunt," another local cunning woman, Sloane MS 1954, §3, 19. She was presumably a real person. The second annotator spells it "Tnugh" in a marginal note, further evidence that these notes are not by Poeton himself.

[35] i.e., pestilence. Current as an adverb as well as a noun at this period, *OED* does not record an adjectival form; however, the meaning is clear (see Gregory's other uses of it, spelled "peslance").

Greg:–: Too tell ee true, I ca-nte tell what too zee toot well, nut I.

Dr:–: I am very glad to see you somwhat relented; I fearde that you had been so firmely fastned unto your owne fantasie: that you woulde not have been at all removed from it, by any strength of reason, or wordes of wisdome; for you were (at the first) peremptorilye pertinacious.

Greg:–: Good Mr Dr: let mee request won thing oye.

Dr:–: Good neighbour: any thing that I can accommodate you in, I will readily yeeld to your request.

Greg:–: Zeeing your gentelnes iz zuch that you wooll doo zo, than I pray, conzidder that I ham a playne cuntry man, an I do-nte understand no vine allegant words, nut I. Wherevore chud intreate your worship that you woulde speak noe moore zuch vine wordes. Vor too tell ee true, I ca-nte tell what too make o-eme nut I.

[19] *Dr*:–: What wordes are these which you understand not?

Greg:–: Marry zur: groaet menny vine wordes whuch cha quite vorgott. But I remember what you zed last: you zed (an you bee rememberd) that chwaz at tha vurst, parmantorily parmitacious, I do-nte know what you meane byte nut I.

Dr:–: Neighbour my meaning was (by those wordes which I spake) that I thought you to have been of that resolute stubborne condition, that I much feared that I shoulde never have fastned any sounde reason uppon you: But I am glad to fynde it otherwayes now. And I trust that for the time to come you are fully and firmly resolved that you will never have recourse to any of those wise woemen agayne.

The common sorte hardly brought to see their errour.

Greg:–: Too tell ee true zur: Ize dee meane too conzidder ote a littell better, avores go too um agen, cha holde a groate ont. But I know nut it, what I shall doo heerafter: vor still mee thinks that the shud nut bee zo bad, az you dee zeem too make um.

Dr:–: Far be it from mee to speake any other thing then truthe of them, or of any of them. And for myne owne parte, I protest that I hate not the person, of any one of them: But shoulde much rejoyce in the conversion of the worst of them. But the end of all my speech is to make you and such as you are, to know, that such kinde of people, are servants unto Sathan, how greate a shew of sanctitie soever they make before the worlde: and to warn you of them that you goe not agen unto them, leaste that you bee further defyled by them. In which respect, as I have heretofore shewed you some severall sortes of Sathans servants, together with the greate esteem that they were in, with many monarchs, Potentates, Princes, and myghty men of this worlde. So now I purpose to shew you their severall sciences, that so you may know them the better: and once knowing them, that you may abhorr their societie for ever.

Greg:–: Pray zur: doo ene az you ha zed: An by the grace of God, chill harken tee, I an mark well what ee ze.

Dr:–: I am glad to fynde so good a resolution in you. Wherefore for method and memorye sake, I wyll first shew you such as I finde to be recorded in holy writt: after that, I will tell you of som other sortes of them: which I have read of in other Authors: together with **[20]** their natures, offices, and imployments. And as for such as I have collected out of holy writt: I will speake of them Alphabettically.[36] Wherefore Ile first begin with *Astrologers*. Which name I fynde sundry times written, in the prophecye of holy *Daniell chap.* 2. *ver.* 2. 10. 27. Likewise *chap.* 5. *ver.* 7. 11. 15. And the name (as sayth the learned) signifieth a *Gazer* on the heavens: a foreteller of things to com; from the cloudes. Theis sortes were mayntayned by: called for: and consulted with: by those two greate kings of *Babylon*, viz. *Nebuchadnezzar: and Belchazzar his sonn.* And the people of Israell were much blamed by holy *Jeremy*: for geving heed unto such *Jeremiah chap.* 27. *ver.* 9. Theis in our dayes are called *Stargazers*. Theis are such as cast nativities: and erect figures, presuming the presageing of future events.

The second sorte are called *Caldeans*: of theis you may likewise reade in the forementioned chapters of holy *Daniell*: Theis were such as sought to discover secrets by *Sathanicall* conjectures.

A third sorte are called *Charmers*. Theis are such as the *Royall* prophett *David* speakes of. Psalms 58. 5. And of these speakes King *Solomon* in *his Ecclesiastes chap.* 10. in *ver.* 11. There are of theis many among us, who have charmes against the biting of Mad dogs. The stinging of serpents. Bleeding at the nose. Blastings. Inflamations. Burnings with fyer. Scalding with water. Agewes. *Toothache. Cramps. Stitches*, prickings, rageings, akeings, swellings,

[36] Listing the different types of magical practitioner named in scripture in this manner was a common technique used by those who wrote about witchcraft. Similar lists or discussions of these terms are provided, for example, by: Scot, *Discouerie*, bks. 6–15; George Gifford, *A Discourse of the subtill Practises of Deuilles by Witches and Sorcerers* (London: for Toby Cooke, 1587), chap. 3; Henry Holland, *A Treatise Against VVitchcraft* (Cambridge: John Legate, 1590), B4^{r}–D4^{v}; Perkins, *Discovrse*, chaps. 3 and 4; Bernard, *A Gvide To Grand-Ivry*, 244–48. The list has its origins in Deuteronomy 18:10–12, later quoted by Poeton.

hart burnings, flowings of the head &c.[37] In like sorte some have charmes, to dryve away Myce, or Ratts. Spells: to preserve a house, feilde, garden, or orchard from the ryott of robbers: or els to detayne such as shall com into them, (as it were in a prison) untill such time as it shall please the *Charmer* to enlarge them.[38] I once knew a Tinker, who had a charme (as I was informed) against Moles, that by his charme hee woulde have caused all the Moles in a feilde, (of what extent soever it were) to com forthe of the grounde, at som certayne hole, which hee woulde open in the earth, hee onely walking the circumference of that feilde, and using his charme (as hee went) and by making certayne crosses on the grounde as hee went: so that if one stoode at the hole which hee had made for the Moles egression, hee mought easily take them up one after another, as they came from foorth the earth. Theis: with sundry the like are the pleasures and practises, of many miserable unsanctified miscreants. And yet theis think, that thereby they doe God service, and their country much good.

[21] A fourthe sorte of the devills disciples, are called Diviners. Such (being in compact with *Sathan*) undertake the foretelling of things to come: of such there is mention made in the second booke of the Kings *chap*. 17. ver. 17.

A fift sorte are called *Enchanters*. Theis are not much differeing from *charmers*, and you may finde them mentioned in the prophecie of *Isaiah*, *chap*. 47. *ver*. 9. in whose dayes they abounded in Israell: neither is England without such. Theis use *charmes*, Spells, &c. and undertake the cure of witchcraft. &c.

A sixt sorte of this societie, are Magicians. Theis (by their art, as formerly hath been spoken) can make thinges seem to the sight, to be otherwise then they are indeed. Of this sorte and sect were *Jannes* and *Jambres*, in Egipt: Who were set on worke by

---

37 Flowings of the head refers to a flow of "humours" or rheum. With thanks to Jennifer Evans.

38 On charms, see: Davies, *Popular Magic*; Jonathon Roper, ed., *Charms and Charming in Europe* (Basingstoke: Palgrave Macmillan, 2004). For a compendium of contemporary examples, see the large number of charms printed by Scot in his *Discouerie*, esp. bk. 12. Included by Scot are charms against the biting of mad dogs, against the toothache, and against agues; see chaps. 14 and 18. Later in the seventeenth century John Aubrey recalled a charm against toothache, used when he was young, which involved wearing a tooth taken from a skull in the churchyard; *Three Prose Works*, ed. John Buchanan-Brown (Fontwell: Centaur Press, 1972), 229.

King *Pharaoh*, to withstand and oppose *Moses* and *Aaron*, as you may reade in the booke of *Exodus*.[39] And I think that some of the Juglers of theis times are their *Apes*, if they be not of their ofspring.

A seventh sort of Sathans servants, are called *Necromancers*. That is, such as consult with the dead. The vulgar counte and call such as theis, by the names of Conjurers, and stile their art, *The black art*. Of theis you may reade, in the booke of *Deuteronomy ch.* 18. *ver.* 11. As also in *Isay ch.* 8. *ver.* 19.[40] Few of theis profess physick, yet I have knowne some of them so to doe. Theis are resorted to, and consulted with, aboute such thinges, as have been lost or stolne.

The eight in order in Sathans Oeconomie: is *Pythoniss*: those of this sort have their familiar spirits by whose help, they geve answeres unto such as resorte unto them, and that concerning things past, present, and to com (But of this doubtfull), Of this sorte and sect, you may finde mention made. *Leviticus* 19. 31. &c. &. 20. 27. *Deuteronomy* 18. 11. & 1. *Samuel* 28. 7. *Isay* 29. 4. *Acts* 16. 16. And of all other the servants of Sathan, theis are the greatest in number, highest in esteem: moste frequented.

The ninthe of this nest: are Soothsayers: theis make som outward profession of art and undertake to tell things from the observation of the heavens, and of the clowdes: from their motions: and from their colours. Theis by *Moses* are called (as our last translation renders it) observers of times.[41] From the following of such: The prophet Jeremy dehorts.[42] *ch.* 27. *ver.* 9.

The tenth of this tribe, I finde to be termed *Wizards*. Theis presume to presage of future events. And of theis you may reade. *Leviticus* 19. 31. *Deuteronomy* 18. 11. &. 1. *Samuel* 28. 9.

Now there are besides all theis, sundry other Magicall arts and sciences, which (amongst the heathen) have been taught by sundry sects of prophane *Philosophers*. Of whom wee may reade in the book intituled *The treasurie of ancient and modern times* **[22]** penned by those worthyes *Pedro Mexio*, a *Spaniard*: *Francescus Sansovinus*, an *Italian*. As also those honourable frenchmen, *Anthonie du Verdier, Lord of Vaupriuaz*: *Loys Guyen, Sieur de la Nauche* counsellor unto the king: *Claudius Gurget Parisian*. &c. and translated into English

[39] Exodus 7:9–12.

[40] i.e., Isaiah.

[41] Poeton refers to the 1611 translation of Deuteronomy 18:10. The Geneva Bible has "regarder of times"; *The Bible* (Geneva: Rouland Hall, 1560).

[42] Counsels against.

Lib. 6. chap. 15.

by one unnamed.[43] Wherefore Ile relate them unto you, in the same order as they are sett downe by our foresayde Authors. And first to begin with *Phisiognomie*, or *Metroposcopy*: which is to divine by the forehead. *Chyromancie*: is to divine by the hand (this art with us is called by the name of *Palmistrye*). *Pyromancye*: is to divine by fire. *Hydromancye*: by water. *Geomancye*: is to divine by pointes throwne at peradventure.

Necromancy or *Necyomancy*: is to divine, by conference with the dead.

Auruspicy: were such as did divine by the flyghts and songs of byrds.

Capnomancy: was to divine by fumes, and smoakes.

Botonomancy: was to divine from hearbes, and by sorcery, to heale diseases with them.

The *Phytonicks*, had spiritts in rings Jewells &c.

Cleronomancy: is a Soothsaying by lotts.

Ichthynomancy: is a divineing by fishes.

Cosinomancy: is a divineing by a Sive. This hath been much used within the compass of my time. Theis with some others say our Authors, are spoken of,[44] by *Prochus*.[45] *Porphyrius*.[46] *Iamblicus*.[47]

---

[43] *The Treasvrie Of Avncient And Moderne Times, Containing the Learned Collections, Iudicious Readings, and Memorable Obseruations: Not onely Diuine, Morrall and Phylosophicall. But also Poeticall, Martiall, Politicall, Historicall, Astrologicall, &c.* (London: William Jaggard, 1613) was an enormous compendium of information on a huge range of topics (as the subtitle suggests); a kind of early encyclopaedia, although without any observable sense in the ordering of the material. This list, which is more detailed in the original, appears in a chapter entitled "Of the sottish and ydle opinions, observed among the Sects of Phylosophers: discouering (briefly) all Sciences, Arts, and Doctrines, with their abuses and vanities." The section referred to by Poeton is at 581–83.

[44] This list is taken verbatim from *The Treasvrie of Avncient And Moderne Times*. These authors, however, would have been thoroughly familiar to educated early modern readers in their own right.

[45] Proclus (c. 410–485), a major Neoplatonist philosopher. The ancient Neoplatonists were strongly engaged in both the practice and defence of ritual magic.

[46] Porphyry (c. 234–c. 305), Neoplatonist philosopher and notable anti-Christian author. His biography of his teacher Plotinus (c. 205–270), founder of Neoplatonism, contains extensive discussion of the latter's magical activities and beliefs.

[47] (c. 250–325), Neoplatonist philosopher who studied under Porphyry and subsequently founded his own school. His *On the Mysteries of*

Colophonius.[48] *Apuleius.*[49] *Cornelius Agrippa.*[50] As also by St Augustine.[51]

Loe neighbour *Gregory*: (as you have heard) I have even harrowed hell (as it were) for your sake: how like you this rabblement? are they not a fayre litter of lewde ones think you? What say you now to our former question: whether (think you) have you sinned against God or not, in your so often going unto your good vokes?

Greg:–: Master doctor, I must ene tell ee true, I ca-nte tell well what too ze toot: I dowt cha zind indeed, God vorgee mee. Indeed I thought that the had been good vokes, zo I did. But now I ca-nte well tell what too think oate, nut I.

Dr:–: Ile advise you think of such, as God thinks of them: and to esteem of them according as God doth esteem of them, and no otherwise.

Greg:–: An pray zur: how doo God steem o zuch vokes?

Egypt is a defence of ritual magic and contains discussions of the invoking of daemons.

[48] Nicander of Colophon (second century B.C.), physician and poet.

[49] (c. 125–c. 180), Roman author and Platonist. His *Metamorphoses* or *The Golden Ass* was a popular work in early modern England; it centres around the protagonist's dabblings in magic. Apuleius was also the author of *De Deo Socratis*, a treatise on the existence and nature of demons, attacked by Augustine, and another work in defence of magic, written when he himself was accused of witchcraft (he was not convicted).

[50] Heinrich Cornelius Agrippa (1486–1535) was a notorious sorcerer, alchemist, and astrologer, among other things. His *Three Books of Occult Philosophy* were enormously influential on subsequent magical writing and were a bête noire for those who wrote against magic.

[51] Augustine of Hippo (354–430) was one of the most important Christian theologians. His major work, *The City of God against the Pagans*, was influential throughout early modern Europe. It contains several discussions of magic and spiritual activity. Augustine's comments on the false distinction between witchcraft and white magic have particular relevance to Poeton's treatise (and are the roots of much of the medieval and early modern attack on popular magic): "Our adversaries try to distinguish certain persons who are devoted to illicit arts, whom they call sorcerers, and who, they say, practise witchcraft, from others who seem to them worthy of praise because they practise theurgy. In truth, however, both classes are equally bound by the false rites of the demons whom they worship under the names of angels." From the translation by R. W. Dyson (Cambridge: Cambridge University Press, 1998), bk. 10, chap. 9, 404. *The Treasvrie Of Avncient And Moderne Times* refers readers to the seventh and eighth books of Augustine's work.

Dr:–: His holy worde wyll make that playne unto you. In regard whereof Ile request of you, dilligently to mark, what is heer written by holy Moses, in the booke called *Deutronomie ch.* 18. *ver.* 10. 11. 12. *There shall not be founde among you, any one that maketh his sonn or his daughter to pass through the fyer,* **[23]** *or that useth diviniations, or an observer of tymes, or an enchanter, or a witch, or a charmer, or a consulter with famylyar spirits, or a wizard, or a Necromancer, for all theis things are an abomination unto the lord: and because of theis abominations, the lord thy God doth dryve them* (that is the heathen) *out before thee.* Neighbour what say you to this?

Greg:–: I can zay littell toot: all at I can zay iz this, mee thinks still, that zuch vokes as doo no harme, shud not bee witches.

Dr:–: Alas neighbour, you consider not the greate hurt that these doe: I feare that you are not as yet capeable thereof: such hurts as are incident unto the bodyes of men and beastes: you are (I dare say) sencible of: but as for many evills, whereby the soule is harmed and hurt, of theis you have scarce any feeling at all. The reason whereof is evident enough, which is, that you are more carnall then spirituall. For were you illuminated from above, you woulde have a greater care of the welfare of your soule, then now you have of the health of your bodye. And then you woulde soone discerne, that such as you affect; coulde not doe what they doe, nor tell what theyle tell, without som asistance from Sathan: I am very sorry to finde you thus inconstant: for but even now you seemed to shew som remorse of conscience, and sorrowe for your sinnes committed against almighty God, in regarde of this, that you had gone unto such people, who worke not by ordynarie, lawfull, and sanctified meanes: but (as you then seemed to conceve it) by som association with Sathan. But answere mee (I pray you) directly; whether doe you think, is the more precious, (and worthy of esteem, respect, and care,) either your soule or your body?

Greg:–: Master doctur, why shud you ax mee such a question? I thong God, cham nut zo verry a voole it, but thats dee think, my zoule too bee better than my boddye.

Dr:–: I am glad that you are so understanding heerin: Now seeing that you acknowledg your soule, to be better then your bodye: you must (in equitie) confess that you ought then to have more care of the welfare of your soule; then of the health of your bodye: and that you ought to prefer the good of your soule, before all the goods of this worlde. According to that saying, of our blessed lord and Saviour. *Matthew* 16. 26. *For what is a man profited, if hee shall gaine the whole worlde and lose his owne soule?*

Greg:–: But I trust in God, that a man shall nut looze his zoule, vor going **[24]** too those vokes, shall a?

Dr:–: Undoubtedly yes: if hee repent not.

Greg:–: Why: ze, that a man dud it of ingrance: wooll God bee zo hard, az too dam won vor that?

Dr:–: Yea if hee repent not, and so gett pardon in Christ. For ignorance will not excuse any man, before Gods just tribunall: As may be gathered from out of the twelth chapter of St *Lukes gospell*: *ver.* 48. And in *Leviticus ch.* 4. *ver.* 2. &c. you may see, that there was a sacrifice appointed for that sin, as well as there were sacrifices for other sinns.

Greg:–: An ta bee zo, than God helps. But won thing chud request oye, Mr doctur: pray tell mee, how shud won know um too be witches? Vor anz did wonce know um, chill zware on a book, that chud nere go too um agen: zo chud nut: nut I.

Dr:–: Neighbour: I am very willing to satisfye your request heer in; and that even unto my utmost abillitie. Wherefore I entreate you, carefully to mark those things which I shall relate unto you. And therefore understand: that.[52]

Rules whereby white witches may be discovered.

First those kinde of people, are (for the most parte) ignorant of the groundes, and rules of all lawfull art: being generally, weake, and unlearned woemen. In which respect, they cannot endure to have any conference with any wise, learned, judicious, or well experienced *Phisition*. And if (by chance) they hap to com where any such are: you shall soone see them as mute as fishes.

Secondly: they are voyde of all soundnes of judgment, in matters of *Pietie*, and as free from sinceritie in matter of practice. In regarde whereof you shall hardly procure any one of them, to confer with a Judicious Divine either concerning the true God: his nature: essence: incommunicable properties: divine attributes: or of his worde, worshipp, and service. Neither can you perswade them to reveale their prayers unto any such.

Thirdly: you shall finde them to be observers of times: as of good and bad dayes, and of lucky and unlucky howers. Yea, you shall finde them to be fraught with supersticious observations: As the crossing of a *Hare*: The falling of salt towards one: The howling

[52] The following list is a slightly modified version of a list given by Richard Bernard in his *A Gvide To Grand-Ivry Men* (1627). Bernard was a prolific author on many religious topics; his witchcraft treatise is largely a compendium of earlier writing on the subject, both English and Continental, but would go on to be influential, both on later authors and on a number of witch trials. To compare Bernard's list, see Appendix.

of doggs: Croaking of Ravens: Crying of the Scrytch Owle: with divers other such like dotages, which they teache Simple people to observe.

Fourthly: they (ordinarily) are greate boasters: magnifying and extolling themselves for art and abillities, to be without compare: by which meanes, they gayne to themselves much creditt and custom, from the common sorte of people.

Fiftly: (in private) they profess themselves, able to help those that are taken (as they terme it) under an ill planet: or such as have undergone the mallice of **[25]** som mischeevous tongue: or such as are bewitched.

Sixtly: some of them wyll desire to have some things brought unto them, which have been worne next unto the body of the person, that sends unto them for counsayle: And having any such thing brought unto them: You shall see them to folde, unfolde: refolde: trefolde: and fowerfolde the same, into sundry fantastick formes, turning it now this way, anon another way: as if those Wizards, woulde measure the fower windes therewith. In all which time, you may perceve them to whisper and mutter softly to themselves.

Seventhly: theyle (sometymes) teach their clyents (who resorte unto them) certayne *Charmes* and *Spells*: which they call prayers.

Eightly: they have not many medicines; for *Varietie* and they, are at variance: And those few which they have, they promiscuously geve, at all times; to all persons: uppon all occasions. Now all wise men know, that the body of many is subject unto a thowsand maladyes: how then can all those so divers and discrepant diseases be cured with so few medicines as theis folkes are furnished withall: yea and oftentimes (as my self can testifie) they geve and appoint meanes and medicines, wholely impertinent unto the cure of the Malady. But what care they, what it is which they either geve or appoint: all that they doe in this case is but to delude the worlde: and to serve them as a mask to vizzor their magick art from the eyes of men: according to that which Mr *Phylomathes* lately related, concerning the confession of the witch of Clare.

A ninthe note of the byrds of this nest; is their prescience or foreknowledg, of such as are to come unto them: as also for whom: for what cause: and at what time.[53] Now who will undertake to

[53] A slightly later example of a white witch supposedly able to predict the purpose of a client's visit is found in Edmond Bower's *Doctor Lamb Revived* (London: Thomas Wilson[?] for Richard Best and John Place, 1653), an account of cunning woman Anne Bodenham's trial for witchcraft in 1652; see page 2. Bodenham's powers in this respect, however,

prove that theis things may be done by lawfull and laudable art: and not rather confess, that such as those, are the schollers and servants of Sathan: and that they are very proficient, bothe in their profession and practice.

A tenth token to know a white Witch by: is their telling who are bewitched: as also how: when: and by whom: Yea and somtimes they will reveale those secret parts, where the devill sucks blood from the black witch. All which they doe by the help of their famylyar spirit.

An eleventh evidence of that infernall art, is, that some of them, at some times, will shew the suspected black witch in a glass. Which thing hath often been related, by sundry such as have resorted unto them.[54]

[26] A twelfth cognisance whereby they may be knowne, is their preventing of such as come unto them for councell: for as I have been credibly informed by some that have been resorters unto them, they have at some times, unto some persons, bothe tolde them from whom and from whence they came, and what their buisines was. And some of those who related these things unto mee, are yet living: and have proffered to depose the truthe and certayntie heerof, whensoever Authoritye shoulde require it.

A thirteenth tryall is, to take this into consideration, that theis sortes of people require credence or confidence in such as resorte unto them: And they will much blame those for diffidence or distrust if they finde it in them: telling such that they can not doe them any good, unless they beleeve well. Thus doe those wicked wretches rob God of his honour: And ruine the soules of such as run a whooring after them.

The last (though not the leaste) note, of a white witch is, that theyle tell (and that) uppon the sole inspection of a carryed urine, what is the state of a sick person, together with all occasions and

are not consistently reliable. Bernard's references (see previous note) are to Alexander Roberts's *Treatise of Witchcraft* (London: Nicholas Okes for Samuel Man, 1616).

[54] The supposed ability of white witches to show the face of the person they suspect has bewitched their client (or that their client suspects has bewitched them) in a variety of surfaces is amply testified to by treatises of the period: see e.g., Gifford, *Dialogve*, B1^{r}, D4^{v}–E1^{r}, E4^{r}; Perkins, *Discovrse*, 208, and see quotation from Bernard in Appendix. Scot suggests that trick glasses, able to show a variety of different things, can be purchased or made; *Disouerie*, 316.

occurrences of the disease whatsoever, and that constantly unto all comers whosoever: which can no way be performed by lawfull art.

Now neighbour *Gregory*: what say you to theis things? Tell mee truely: have you not at some time or other, observed some of theis former marks, badges, signes, tokens, or evidences of white Witchcraft, in some of those wise folkes that you have so often resorted to? Answere mee what think you of them now?

Greg:–: Think ome: marry zur: I know nut what too think ome, nut I. That whuch you ha now e zed, (I may tell you) it ha put mee too zuch a peslance purdicament, that I know nut (in all tha worlde) what too ze toot. An too tell ee true, I donte like um hafe zo well az chwaz woont too doo. Alas ee may zee what ingrant people, wee playne country vokes bee that ha no lurning. I did nere think till now, that all tha men in tha worlde coud ha zed hafe zo much agen um, az you ha now e zed. An vor my parte (chee tell ee true) I did think that the had e ben az good voke, az enny boddy shud ha cum too house too. God vorgee mee vor going zo oft too um: It chill zware on a booke, that I thought no harme int. But vor this trick alone, chill nere goe too enny ome agen, zo I wonte, nut I. Vor an ere I shud ha need agen: chill goe too a *Vizichian*, though cham shure avore hond, that my purse must pay well vort.

[27] *Dr*:–: Neighbour: I am very glad to see this so happy a change in you: geve almighty God the glorye of your inlightning; by whose grace you are come to see your error. And I pray the same God to perfect what hee hath begun in you.

Greg:–: Indeed master doctur, I thank you with all my hart, vor your good will. An chill promise you won thing, that chill zend you tha vats pigg that I ha, whon somever youle pointe too have zent tee. But pray zur (if zo bee that I may speake without any fence tee) doo zo much as tell mee won thing.

Dr:–: Tell mee what that one thing is, which you woulde know of mee.

Greg:–: Why zunce ee are zo gentle: pray donte you think that there bee zum lurnd men that dee deale with tha d'vle?

Many greate persons, have been white witches.

Dr:–: Yes undoubtedly: there (bothe) have been and are such: the greater is their sin; and the heavier will be their judgment. And for your further satisfaction, I wyll tell you of some greate ones, as also of some learned ones, who have had association with Sathan: And first to begin with *Manasseh* king of *Judah*: (the sonn of good King *Hezekiah*) hee used Inchantments, and dealt with familiar spirits, and Wizards &c. As wee may reade in the second booke of the Kings *ch.* 21. *ver.* 6. To passe by *Symon Magus* (of whom wee have formerly spoken) who bewitched the people of Samaria with his Sorceries. *Acts* 8. 9. *Eusebius* in his ecclesiasticall history,[55] makes mention of one *Manes* an *Heritick* who (by the power of *Sathan*) mounted himself up into the *Ayre*, in the presence of a greate number of people, flying quite out of their sight. And in the same history, hee sayth that *Maxentius*, *Maximinus*, and other Emperours: used Magicall arts: And that those Emperours woulde admitt no Governours, Captaines or Officers, but such as were instructed therein. Neither woulde they advance or prefer any but such as were skild in that science. Againe, *Platina* (in his booke of the lives of the Popes,) affirmeth that Pope *Sylvester* the second: as also *Joane* the Papess obtayned the Romane primacy by art *Magick*.[56] And St Augustine (in his ninthe booke of the Citie of God) speakes of many such, whom he knew to be skild in that cursed science.[57] And *Marcus Varro*: speakes marvelous thinges of the transforming of men into beastes: who after some certayne yeares, returned unto their pristine state and shape agayne.[58] I have likewise read of one Circes an Enchantress who transformed the companions of *Ulisses* into swine, by meanes of a certayne drink which shee gave them.[59]

---

[55] Eusebius, Bishop of Caesarea (c. 260–c. 340), scriptural commentator and ecclesiastical historian. There were several English editions of his *Ecclesiastical Histories* available to Poeton. On Manes (founder of the Manichean heresy), see the first English edition (London: Thomas Vautroullier, 1577), bk. 1, chap. 17; although the text names Manes as a sorcerer, I have been unable to find reference to his powers of flight. On Maxentius and Maximinus, see bk. 8, chaps. 15 and 16.

[56] Bartolomeo Sacchi, known as Platina (1421–1481) was an Italian humanist. His *Vitæ Pontificum* was first published in 1479. There were no English editions published during Poeton's lifetime, but he could easily have had access to a Continental edition. Pope Sylvester II and Pope Joan (John VIII) were both said by Platina to have obtained the pontificate through "ill arts," i.e., black magic; see the first English translation, *The Lives Of The Popes*, trans. Paul Rycaut (London: for Christopher Wilkinson, 1685), 194 and 165. Pope Joan is a mythical character, but was believed to be real during the early modern period.

[57] On Augustine's *City of God*, see above, note 51.

[58] Marcus Terentius Varro (116–27 BC), Roman poet, satirist, antiquarian, geographer, and grammarian, whose works only survive in fragments. The accounts he gives of human to animal transformation are cited by Augustine, *City of God*, bk. 18, chap. 17. On animal transformation, see below, note 62.

[59] Circe is the sorceress from Homer's *Odyssey*, bk. 10, ll. 233–43; see also Ovid, *Metamorphoses*, bk. 14. Taking examples from imaginative literature as if they were real was a common practice among early modern writers, particularly those who sought evidence of magical practice. Con-

And credible reports have brought it unto our eares, that the greatest part of their religious men among the Turkes are Enchanters and Magicians: and that they bothe doe and tell strange thinges; thereby drawing the people to geve the more **[28]** creditt unto their *Mahometane sect.* And I doubt not but that you have heard of Dr *Faustus* (a doctor of divinitie) of *Wittenberg* in *Germanie,*[60] who gave himself unto the devill bothe body and soule (writing the covenant with his owne blood) for the enjoying the service of a Sathanicall spirit (one called *Mephostophiles*) by the space of xxiiii yeares. There is a booke yet extant of the severall passages thereof.[61] I coulde name sundry of this our owne nation (who have lyved within the compass of my time) who because they were never convict of witchcraft in their lyfe time, I think it good to conceale their names being dead.

This story, I heard to be justified for a truthe by S. of the States of Holland, at the table of Collonell Dyer.

Greg:–: Lord ha marcy uppons all: theis bee strange things indeed, az ere I hurd zunce tha time that chwaz e bore: But won thing, I dee moore marle at than all tha rest: whuch iz, that the shud turne men into beastes. An you had nut e zed it, shure I shud nere ha beeleevd it.

Dr:–: Neither doe I beleeve that they were really and indeed turned into beastes: But I rather think (with St *Augustine*) that they were none other than Sathanicall Illusions.[62]

---

tinental demonologists did so regularly, and although the practice was less widespread among English authors, they too had recourse to classical sources when they felt the need. See for example Perkins, *Discovrse*, 197; Roberts, *Treatise*, 8–9 and *passim*; Cotta, *The Infallible Trve And Assvred Witch*, 39, 42. Reginald Scot complained about the practice in scathing terms, picking on earlier authors' use of this very example; see *Discouerie*, bk. 12, chap. 8, 229.

60 Marginal note: I have been unable to identify these figures. Dyer was a relatively common name in Sussex during the period.

61 Poeton presumably refers to the prose narrative of Faustus's life rather than Marlowe's play (for which the former was the main source). *The Historie of the damnable life, and deserved death of Doctor Iohn Faustus* is first known to have been translated into English by the mysterious P. F. and published in London in 1592; a reissue appeared in 1622 and a new edition in 1636. See John Henry Jones, ed., *The English Faust Book* (Cambridge: Cambridge University Press, 1994).

62 On the transformation of humans into animals by the power of witches, Poeton is in agreement with his fellow authors of treatises on witchcraft in England, who widely rejected the possibility. See for example Gifford, *Dialogve*, K3^{r}; Perkins, *Discovrse*, 27, 33. French demonologist Jean Bodin, whose work was well-known in England, believed that

Greg:–: I dee think zo too. But pray Mr Dr: tell mee won thing moore: it: how doo the doo too get tha d'vle at vurst?

Dr:–: Truely neighbour, I ingeniously confess, that I am not well able to resolve you therein: neither doe I either long or labour to understand it. But tell mee, what moves you to desyre the knowledg thereof?

Greg:–: Indeed zur vor no hurt in all tha worlde nut I: it (vor all that) chud vayne knowte: Mee thinks ans knew but that, twood zatisvy my minde very much: I, an yease my stummack abomynably well.

Phy:–: May it please Mr doctor to geve mee leave. Ile tell you somthing that I have knowne concerning that which hee requests.

Greg:–: Marry zur: Wood you wood bee zo gentle. I know that Mr Dr is zuch a good man that hee wooll gee ee leave, zo a wooll.

Dr:–: Yes indeed, with all my hart.

Greg:–: How zay now Mr *Phymolathes*? Mr Dr (I thank him) zayes that heel gee ee leave, wee alls hart. Wherevore praye ze what you know in this matter: I can tell ee, ta may doo mee, an zuch az I am, more good than you ar aware on, zoet may.

Phy:–: Seeing that you are so desyrous to heare what I shall be able **[29]** to say concerning this matter, I faythfully promise you that I will not spare to speake, that which I know herein: although (in some sorte) I shall thereby discover some of myne owne faults and fraylties. But let God have due glory: let his people have the benefit: and let mee beare myne owne deserved blame.

Thauthors free confession.

Greg:–: Well vare your good hart zur: vor ee speake leek an onnest man. An vor that trick, chill promize ee won thing: Chill mark well what ee zay: An I hope twooll doo mee good. An cha tell ee

such transformations were a real possibility, but his views were not widely accepted by his fellow authors on the subject; see *On the Demon-Mania of Witches*, trans. Randy A. Scott (Toronto: Centre for Reformation and Renaissance Studies, 2001), bk. 2, chap. 6. Examples of this supposed power are occasionally found in the pamphlet literature of the period, suggesting that there may have been a level of popular belief in the possibility. See for example *A Rehearsall both straung and true, of hainous and horrible actes committed by Elizabeth Stile, Alias Rockingham, Mother Dutten, Mother Deuell, Mother Margaret, Fower notorious Witches, apprehended at winsore* (London: [John Kingston] for Edward White, 1579), A5^{r}; Thomas Potts, *The Wonderfvll Discoverie Of Witches In the Covntie of Lancaster* (London: William Stansby for John Barnes, 1613), K4^{v}–L1^{r}, L2^{r}. For Augustine's comments on the subject, see *The City of God*, bk. 18, chap. 18.

true, that cham glad wee all my hart that twaz my good vortune too meet zo luckely wee ee heere.

Phy:–: Well: since you have so freely and frendly exprest your minde, in desiring satisfaction in this matter. Ile therefore presently pitch uppon the pointe: and without any manner of either circumstance or circumlocution, (more then necessitie shall enforce) I will intentionally prosecute the matter in hand, and that with as much perspecuitie and playnenes, as the subject will permitt, and my poore abilities extend unto.

Greg:–: Mr *Phymolathes*: in my poore zimple pinnion, yo ze zo much az enny onnest man in tha worlde can ze: An too tell ee true, vor my parte I shall nere counte him a onnest man that wood dezire moore of a man, than hees able vor too doo.

Phy:–: Well: not to trifle away our precious time with any more impertinent prattle. Honest frend: I request you advisedly to heed, what I shall deliberately declare unto you. Understand therefore that the devill is that Arch sublunary inspector of nature, cautiously considering, all Agents and actions whatsoever: knowing more of natures secrets, then all the wise of the worlde, either doe or can, without speciall Illumination from the moste high. But his cheef imployment is to compass and consider mankinde, whose ruine is his repaste; whose destruction is his delight: and whose perdition, hee perpetually plotteth. Yea it is even hee, of whom St *Peter* forewarneth Christians to be carefull and cautelous to arme themselves against, in his first epistle, *ch.* 5. *ver.* 8. Now *Sathan*: thus constantly compassing: thus carefully considering mankinde: when hee espies any one (whether male or female) over eagerly to affect, Science and *Knowledg* beyond modest measure: then will hee labour without delay: by som slyght or stratagem, to insinuate himself into them. The which to effect, hee wanteth **[30]** neither will nor skyll, art nor industry: hee hath a storehouse full of sleyghtes, stratagems, and snares: which hee is able to manage (for his owne advantage) at all times, in all places, against all persons. So that there is neither man nor woman, if they be not kept by the keeper of Israell: but that they are sure to be caught by this subtill Soule hunter: for hee knowes each ones constitution: hee dyves into eache severall disposition: eyes eache inclination: and fishes out eache affection: and accordingly tempers all his temptations. For hee can (*Proteus* like) change himself into all colours, formes and fashions: heele propose honour, to the ambitious: wealth, to the covetuous: pleasures, to the voluptuous: the knowledge of hidden secrets, unto the curious: In a worde, hee hath snares for every sence, by which hee entraps the poore soule.

But to passe by all the rest, and to speake simply and solely concerning that, which hath hitherto been (and still is) the subject of our present discourse, to wit: how or by what meanes men and woemen com to have asociation with Sathan, I submissively shew my poore opinion therein: when *Sathan* sees any one, desirous of knowledg above the boundes of mediocrytie; then hee useth all his infernall art, to exasperate that desyre: and accordingly as hee findes them to be furnished, either with naturall endowments: or any measure of supernaturall grace, so will hee insinuate into them; or make som onset uppon them: for put the case, that some meane simple *Schollar* gett some booke or bookes of *Chyrurgery*: and with some dilligence doe reade and study the same; and from thence shall rush uppon practice, without sounde judgment: and so be put to a *Non plus* at his greatest need; then will the devill use all dilligence to put an edge to his appetite, and to enflame his affections, with a fervent desyre, to attayne som exquisite measure of excellency in art. And now if the devill finde him to be weake in, (or voyde of) fayth: then will hee boldely present himself unto him, with tender of his service uppon certayne covenants and condicions twixt them to be agreed uppon. But if Sathan see in them, any fruites of fayth, or finde that they have any measure of sounde knowledg, then heel take some other course, as by his suggestions, to send them to some of his former sworne servants, who shall (by his instigation) geve them free and frendly entertaynement: and by theis his artificiall agents hee will animate them unto a greater desyre of knowledg which those Impes of Sathan will perswade unto, as being easye in the attayning, and that it will prove, bothe pleasing and profitable in the use. Theis things spur on, to hasten the attaynement of the meanes, whereby this sounde science **[31]** (so much sought for) may be attayned: which must be by getting the asosiation of an Angell (at the leaste) who woulde further him more in knowledg in one yeare, then any universitie coulde doe in a whole age. And loe: by theis kinde of courses and proceedings, is there (by this time) a fyre kindled within the entrayles of this curious searcher after knowledg, that if it be not quenched (with the water that flowes from out of the fountayne of life) it will burne as deep as hell.

Greg:–: Now well vare your good hart: ee had zed verre well too tha purpose indeed. But pray wooll ee bee zo gentle az too goe on: cham zorry that chwaz zo voolish az too tarrupt ee in your talke.

Phy:–: Honest frend: theres no cause of sorrow in the matter: for I have gayned a good breathing time by the bargayne. But to proceed: such as (in this case) are left unto themselves, once hearing of such an easy and short way, to attayne unto such a height of excellent knowledg: and that not onely in *Chyrurgery*, (before named) but also in *Physick* much more to be desyred, they seldome goe back, or delay, any time; but with all possible expedition: get themselves into that same Soule Slaying Societie. And now to come to a free confession of myne owne faults and follyes (geving *Almighty God* the glory, of his mercy and goodnes towards mee): So it was that aboute the Aprill of myne age even when my veynes ran full of blood: my bones were fild with marrow: and my whole body, vigorously abounding with vitall spirits, I then much desyred the knowledg of Arts, and that with (no les) than an exorbitant eagernes. And being somwhat impatient of the paines of study: I thought with my self that there mought be som nearer way founde out (for the attayning of what I desyred) then laboriously earely and late to be plodding at my booke. Whereuppon in short space I occasionally came acquainted, with two men; very famous for their excellent skill in their art: bothe of them being profest, and alowed *Physitions*: I founde their houses much frequented: their persons much reverenced: their skill applawded: and themselves (by greate ones) often imployed. By bothe of these, I was courteously entertayned, and had free access unto them, and often private parlee, with them. After some small time had passed from our first acquaintance, I then made knowne unto either of them, my desires and intentions: which were by either of **[32]** them, bothe approved and applawded. And they bothe (severally) did prophecy very happy success unto mee in all such myne undertakings and proceedings. And either of them solicited mee to lyve with him for seven yeares, and that not uppon any servile condition: but proffered compainionship unto mee, with a moste free and full revelation of all secrets whatsoever appertayning unto that their Science. And the more to alure mee thereto, and the faster to tye mee thereby; either of them proffered unto mee a daughter in marriage: with a fayre portion of outward estate. Thus was I besett with enemyes on every side; Corrupt nature within: The devill, the world, and the flesh without.[63]

Dr:–: I asure you, that (in mine opinion) you were in a very greate strayght: I pray you to tell the manner of your deliverance, that so wee may magnifie the mercyes of God together with you.

Phy:–: Right worthy Sir: That God (who onely is the true God) who tooke *Moses* out of the waters: delyvered *Danyell* from the Lyons: and the three children from the fyerie fornace:[64] hee, even hee delyvered mee: And his mercy to mee ward is no les marvelous

[63] See introduction for a discussion of this episode.

[64] Exodus 2:1–10, Daniel 6 and 3.

then it was to them: but rather in myne owne apprehension much more: for their delyverances were but from a temporarye death: but myne was from an everlasting destruction both of body and soule. Those were by violence, enforced to what they suffred, or were in danger of. But alas I, (wretched I) voluntarily rusht into the midst of so many mighty and malicious enemies. Those willingly offered up their lyves unto the death for the glory of God. But I (foole that I was) sought to get glory to my self. And yet did the Lord delyver mee, yea even when that I was compassed rounde aboute with those deadly snares. I confess, that the society of those men, was to mee a solace. The meanes, or portion which either of them proffered; was as tempting a bayte, as was *Achans* golden wedg.[65] Their daughters which they tendered: were worthy (in all outward respects) much to be embraced. But the mayne, was that hidden mysterie of iniquitie; the secrets of their science; that was it which my soule thirsted after: for to beholde how they woulde canvase, a carryed urine, and from its bare inspection (as I thought) tell the whole state of a sick person, as readily and as perfectly, as if they had been constantly with him, from the very first time that his sicknes invaded him. This of all the rest seemed moste strange unto mee: because I was then spiritually blinded, and coulde not **[33]** discerne of the truthe. Heeruppon I endevoured to endeare my selfe the more into the men. And as myne occasions permitted, and opportunity served, I more frequently visited them, somtimes thone, somtimes thother. Now their dwellings (at that time) were well neare, fiftie myles asunder. But yet they differed far more in their dispositions from one another, then they were distant in their dwellings. For the one of them (with whom I was first acquainted) was very pleasant and affable, woulde take his cupps, and sweare like a Courtier: yea embrace a curtezan (if hee belyed not himself). But the other, was a man grave in his government, austere in his life, upright and honest in his conversation: and withall very close and reserved. At the first, myne occasions offered mee more frequent recourse unto the former: whose freenes unto me, made mee the more forward, to open my hart unto him: wherefore I emboldened my self to ask of him, how hee attayned that his skill, (seeing that hee was a man well neare illiterate, if not altogether) and how one that was but a meane Scholler mought attayne the like? To this hee answered mee (in short) that it coulde not be attayned without the association of an Angell. But hence grew the doubte: the difficultie how

[65] Joshua 7.

this association with an Angell mought be attayned. Concerning this doubte, hee resolved mee, that it must be by getting and using the Vocabula (as hee calde it) which done, the Angell woulde appeare; attend: afforde assistance, direction, instruction, in what thing soever desired.[66] I then desired to know that Vocabula what it was; but for the present faylde of what I then desired: neither coulde I ever obtayne it from of the masters of those mysteries, but in proces of time I gate the sight and survay thereof; from one of their disciples.

Dr:–: Mr *Phylomathes*: I pray you tell mee what that Vocabula was.

Phy:–: *Reverend Sir*: to speake truthe unto you: It was a meere diabolicall adjuration: charme: or spell: not onely superstitious, (as being interlaced, with sundry crosses and characters) but also fearefully blasphemous: for the sacred names, titles, and attributes, of the most high and most glorious God, were therein moste irreligiously prophaned:[67] And it was penned in parchment (yea if I mistake not, in that, which they call virgin parchment[68]). But the very remembrance thereof makes my very hart to tremble: although for the present (such was my sinn) that I rather tooke pleasure therein. Although (for myne owne parte) I coulde never cause any of their Angels to appeare: by my **[34]** reading thereof.

Dr:–: What were the wordes of that their *Vocabula*?

---

[66] The belief that magicians had the power to summon and converse with angels was widespread among those who credited the occult arts. Opponents of magic believed the spirits to be real; the issue was that they were devils rather than angels (as Poeton goes on to suggest). See introduction.

[67] Vocabula literally means words or names. I have been unable to identify a specific magical text which uses this title, although it is clearly a grimoire of some kind. There were many such works circulating in manuscript in England during this period. See Owen Davies, *Grimoires: A History of Magic Books* (Oxford: Oxford University Press, 2009).

[68] As the name suggests, this is parchment that has not previously been used for anything else, but in ritual magic there is more to it than this. The popular grimoire *Clavicula Salomonis*, a key text in the practice of angelic ritual magic, includes a chapter with instructions on how to prepare virgin parchment. It specifies that it must come from a male animal who has not yet reached sexual maturity, and that certain rituals must be performed both at the slaughtering of the animal and during the subsequent preparation of the parchment. See *The Key of Solomon the King*, trans. and ed. S. Liddell MacGregor Mathers (San Francisco: Weiser Books, 2000), bk. 2, chap. 17. On the *Clavicula*, see Davies, *Grimoires*.

Phy:–: I thank the Lord, I have quite forgotten: And I desyre, never to see, heare, or reade them agayne. And I beseech God (of his goodnes) to keepe mee, and all his, from all those wayes and workes of wickednes.

Greg:–: Marry zur: I cante blame ee, tiz a vearvull thing (I ma tell you) too ha enny thing too doo with tha d'vle: Chea tell ee truely (in my zimple pinnion) God blest ee well: vor ee weare in a peslance purdicament: ee wore beezet on ery zide. Too zee what God can doo: too tell ee true, dee ene maze mee too think ont.

Phy:–: *Oh frend*: had not God been on my side when I was thus besett: I had even perrished in my very prime.

Greg:–: *Shure* an zo ee had indeed: twaz a marlous marcy a God towards ee indeed. But anz may bee so bolde, pray tell mee, how ee did scape?

Phy:–: Ile tell you how: Being on a time solicited by that man, (whom er whiles I mentioned) to entertayne his large (and seeming loving) proffers, it pleased God (of his goodnes) to worke in mee a sodayne dislyke, of his familiar spirit (which hee called his Angell) who (as hee sayde) woulde com being called: for it was geven mee to think, that his familiar was som deceitfull deluding devill. Which conceite I forth with made knowne unto him. But hee woulde fayne have shifted it of, with a bolde asseveration: affirming that hee was moste certayne that it was an holy Angell, which God had geven him for his guardian, guide, and conductor. Yea: further, hee confidently affirmed that hee was the holy Angel *Uriell*, whom God (in olde time) sent unto the prophet *Esdras* 2. *Esdras* 4. 1.[69] And hee audaciously avouched, that his Angell woulde manifest or reveale unto him, what ever hee required of him. And for proofe thereof, hee presently proffered, to shew me instantly, in what place the king of *France* then was, as also what hee was doing: or (in a worde) what els I desyred either to see or know. But it pleased Almighty God, so to enlighten mee (instantly) with his grace, that I grew so to distaste and detest his wordes and wayes, that I utterly refused all that which hee had proffered. And seriously considering his manners and conversation, I founde them to be bothe faulty and foule. As for his wordes and oathes they seemed to mee to be full fraught with vayneglorious ostentation. And I sodaynely saw in them, a

---

[69] The books of Esdras are among the apocryphal books of the Bible. Uriel (2 Esdras 4:1) is a name commonly found in angelic ritual magic from the period; Uriel was among, for example, the angels supposedly summoned by both Dee and Napier. See Raymond, *Milton's Angels*, 107–9, 112.

seeming contradiction: for whereas hee sayde, that hee coulde (and that *ad placitum*[70]) commande that Angell, whom **[35]** God sent unto holy *Esdras*: Mee thought then, that betwixt Gods sending of his holy Angell (and that but once) unto his holy prophet (and that after his greate humiliation: long fasting, and fervent praying) to comfort him. And that this man, (whom I knew to be wicked and prophane) shoulde commande the sayde Angell at his pleasure: Theis things, I assured my self coulde no way stand together, neither in reason, ne yet in religion. Now having thus revolved theis meditations in my minde, after a littell space I proposed the effect thereof unto him: in playne termes telling him that I thought him to be much deluded heerein: saying unto him, that if hee did not apologize the better from himself that then I shoulde instantly fall from him, and utterly forsake him.

Not long before this, I had read that history of the prophet Esdras.

Dr:–: How digested hee that speech of yours?

Phy:–: Surely Sir: I founde it as unwelcom to him, as it was unexpected by him: And at first hee thought to have borne mee quite over with his wayghtles wordes: impudently avouching that his Angell was that very Angell, which God sent unto holy *Esdras*. But to wrest him from his violence, I gan to reason the matter with him, in the mildest manner that I coulde. Speaking either in theis, or some other such like termes. Sir: I pray you answere mee mildely in this: did you ever reade in holy writt, that any man, whether *Patriarch*: *Prophett*: *Apostle*: *Sainte*: or any other servant of God, had any such priveledg (as you boaste of) to commande the service of any of the holy Angels of Almighty God?

Dr:–: What answere coulde hee frame to that your question?

Phy:–: His answere was very poore: viz. that hee had seldome been conversant in the scriptures. And therefore hee was not able from thence to prove, that any man had such a priviledg. But (all that not withstanding) hee for his part, had that happines; hee thankt his God for it. I then desyred him to yeelde mee som reason of that his confidence: whereunto hee answered that the glorious appearance of his Angell unto him, had long since confirmd him in that his conceite. To this I answered, that this was no firme foundation to builde uppon; especially in this so wayghty a buisines, as is the welfare, or ruine of our soules. For: (God permitting) Sathan is able to transforme himself into the likeness of an Angell of light. Sundry other Queres I propounded unto him: but in **[36]** truthe his answeres, were bothe shallow and slyght. At last I askt him of what

[70] As he pleased.

regiment his angell was; and soone perceived that this Quere vext him more than all the rest, for this toucht his tenure to the quick, so that hee seemed not to understand what I meant thereby. But in conclusion, I (by Gods gracious assistance) drave him to this issue, that hee confest, that indeed hee thought it was none of the heavenly Angels; But hee woulde in no case acknowledg that it was a devill, but founde out a fayre *Medium* twixt two extremes: wherewith hee certaynely thought (for ever) to have silenced mee. For hee tolde mee that his *famyliar* was a greate prince of the *Fayries.*[71] To this; I boldely (though somthing unreverently) answered: I think that you are no better then a greate foole so to think. And so for that tyme wee parted, neither ever, was any parle that past betweene us from that day forward.

Dr:–: Undoubtedly, you were much bounden unto Almighty God, for his greate mercyes towards you heerin. But how scapte you the hands of that other man: who was (as you sayde) a man of an austere life?

Phy:–: Doubtles (Sir) if this had not first happened (in all likelyhood) I had been the more entangled. For hee was a man well furnished with Negative vertues: hee was neither Swearer: *drinker*: *Babler*: *Boaster*: or any way prophane in his conversation: but on the contrary hee woulde reprove those sinnes in others. And withall

---

[71] This phrase is underlined, in what looks like the same ink as the secondary annotations, which comment in the margin: "O Ridiculous." Belief in fairies seems to have been widespread in early modern England, though the majority of people were probably ambivalent on the subject. Occasionally elements of the belief cropped up in witch trials, usually in connection with cunning folk who claimed fairies as the source of their power. See Thomas, *Religion and the Decline of Magic*, chap. 19, esp. 727; Peter Marshall, "Protestants and Fairies in Early Modern England," in C. Scott Dixon, Dagmar Freist, and Mark Greengrass, eds., *Living with Religious Diversity in Early Modern Europe* (Farnham: Ashgate, 2009); Peter Marshall, "Ann Jeffries and the Fairies: Folk Belief and the War on Scepticism in Later Stuart England," in Angela McShane and Garthine Walker, eds., *The Extraordinary and the Everyday in Early Modern England: Essays in Celebration of the Work of Bernard Capp* (Basingstoke: Palgrave Macmillan, 2010). There are known cases in which fraudulent cunning folk used fairy lore to cozen their clients: see e.g., *The Brideling, Sadling and Ryding, of a rich Churle in Hampshire, by the subtill practise of one Iudeth Philips, a professed cunning woman, or Fortune teller* (London: T.C. to be sold by William Barley, 1595); *The seuerall Notorious and levvd Cousnages of Iohn West, and Alice West, falsely called the King and Queene of Fayries* (London: for Edward Marchant, 1613).

hee was held to be a good *Scholler*, a master of Arts of many yeares standing. Besides hee had very good success in many greate cures which hee undertooke. Likewise he was very close and reserved. Theis things (considered) wrought in mee a very reverend regarde of the man: And his courteous carriage towards mee, together with his kinde entertayneing of mee, did even captivate myne affections towards him agayne. His wife (likewise) behaved herself like a grave matron: And his daughter (with whom hee tempted mee) had noe fault merriting rejection.

His deep reservednes, sharpned my desyres: whence I was eagerly egd on, to use the meanes whereby I mought attayne, (in some measure) the knowledg of the mysteryes of that his art. But hee like a skilfull master of defence, kept mee still at distance (uppon the poynt) so that I coulde not gett within him without som evident perrill: for unless that I **[37]** woulde covenant with him for certayne society: and becom his son in law, I must still remayne *Statu quo prius.*[72] Theis things did bothe puzzell and pester mee: for I disliked not the bayte, but I dreaded the hooke, though as yet I saw it not. But uppon this, I ceaste to solicite him any further, and bethought my self of a safer course. And instantly entred the search of a more shallow streame, which (as I conceived) flowed from forthe that deep foarde: viz. his man, into whose affection, I screwed my self as close as I coulde: And from him I (gradually) fysht some certayne secrets of that his Masters science. For hee (beeing more simple, and less subtill then his master) shewed mee a prayer, geven him by his master (daily) to use which in effect was, that God (of his goodnes) woulde vouchsafe him the association of one of his holy Angels, to instruct, informe, and assist him. This prayer (as hee confest) hee had long used, and yet had hee never founde any fruite thereof. Then gan I further to enquire; whether that were the sole meanes that his master had ministred unto him, for obtayning of that angelicall association? Heeruppon hee ingeniously revealed the whole truthe unto mee: and shewed mee a long parchment rowlle furnished with sundry crosses and characters: with the names of many Angells (as hee calde them) with severall *Vocabulaes*: (or rather conjurations) tedious to treate of, and terrible to think on. Hee likewise shewde mee a fayre *Crystall stone*, in the which, the spirit (being called) shoulde appeare: and from thence speake in an audible voyce, or els make demonstration of things

[72] In the previous state (i.e., "as I was before").

required. &c.[73] Heeruppon I demanded of him, if at any time hee had seen any such apparition? Whereunto hee answered that hee had not that gift as yet. But hee tolde mee, that hee was promised that hee shoulde have it er long: but hee was to be brought unto it by Circle. Now this speech of his, did strike a kinde of terror into mee, causing some troubled thoughts, to boyle within my breast: but I concealde them to my self, leaste that otherwise, I mought foolishly frustrate my self, in what I desyred to fish from out this fellow. Wherefore I (mildely) askt him, what forme was to be used in that Scene? Unto this hee answered, that as yet, hee never had seen it acted, but the manner thereof had been related unto him by one (who dwelt in *Beech lane*[74]) that had been brought to sight in the Circle. Which was as followeth: viz. The person desirous of the afore sayde angelicall association, was to stand in a convenient place (thereto appoynted) **[38]** and that then, a circle was to be made rounde aboute him, by a master of that Science: with certayne crosses and characters thereon formed: which done, that then there was a white hasell wand (of one yeares growthe) with that moste glorious name (as I remember) *Jehovah*, engraven on the greate end thereof, to be delyvered into his hand (who then stoode within the circle) which hee was to holde still in his right hand, for the use heerafter to be specified. This being done: Then the master was to reade certayne *vocabulaes*, and to use sundry other ceremonyes: which being performed, that then (as hee sayde) the Angels woulde visibly appeare rounde aboute the circle. But beholde: for every holy angell that appeared, there woulde likewise a devill appeare in the same forme. Heeruppon, I demanded of him, how they were to be distinguished? whereunto hee answered, that that (as hee was informed) was to be done by the person, who stoode in the circle: who was to try eache particuler, by tendring unto him, the engraven end of his rod for to kisse, which (as hee sayde) the good Angells (with all reverence) woulde performe: but the evill spirits, woulde turne away their faces. And woulde not in any wise endure the presence of that charactered rod or wand. Heereuppon the person in the circle

[73] Summoning a spirit to appear in a crystal is known as scrying. It was the process used by Dee in his conversations with angels, but the practice was a common element of magical lore, and instructions on how to summon a spirit in this manner are very often found in grimoires from the period (and indeed beyond it). Scot provides an example of just such a ritual; *Discouerie*, bk. 15, chap. 16.

[74] A street in the northern outskirts of London, just outside the city boundary, running west off Whitecross Street, just north of Cripplegate.

made his choyce of that Angell which was moste amiable in his eyes: who ever after woulde attend him. Then I demanded of him, what covenant or contract, then past between that Angell and the new made Artist (or rather Augurist)? To which hee answered, that hee was not informed of any; further then this, viz. that whensoever that artist shoulde call his Angell: that then his Angell woulde appeare unto him, and accommodate him, according to his desyres.

Dr:–: I pray you tell mee, how did this pretty project please you?

Phy:–: Certes Sir: the discovery pleased mee very well: but as for the passages of the pointe, I utterly dislike them, adjudging them to be moste absurd and impious: for I coulde not apprehend it to be otherwise than a meere diabolicall devise, and a Sathanicall stratagem.

Dr:–: Certaynely you are infinitely bounden unto Almighty God who preserved you in the midst of so many perrills. But now by the way, let us pause awhile, and heare what my neighbour *Gregory* thinks of theis things. Neighbour what think you of this last which Mr *Phylomathes* related?

Greg:–: Think oate, I cante well tell what too think oate nut I. Vor too tell ee true, I nere hurd zuch a thing, zunce that time that chwaz vurst e **[39]** bore: But now (vor my parte) chill warrant ee that none onne all shall ere get mee into a zurcle vor this trick: vy uppont, whoo wood ere a thought that enny boddy shud bee made zo verre a voole, az too bee brought too stand in a zurcle, an too ha zo menny d'vles brought aboute um. Theres a mad trick indeed: too tell ee true, dee amoste make mee aveard too think ote. But vor my parte, (an grace a God) vrom hence vorward, chill bee shure too ze my prayers every morning whanz dee rize: I: an sarve God all tha de after. An than I hope God wooll bless mee vrom tha d'vle. An won thing moore chill veth vully promis ee: that chill nere goe no moore to enny o theise wise vokes agen: zo I woante, nut I.

Dr:–: Tis well sayde (of you) Neighbour, doe so indeed and God will bless you. But now Mr *Phylomathes*, I pray you proceed in your discourse.

Phy:–: After those passages (formerly spoken of) I dilligently enquired of him, whether hee knew of any, that had attayned unto that Angelicall association: either by his masters meanes, or by the art of any other?

Dr:–: And what did hee answere unto that your inquisition?

Phy:–: Hee tolde mee of a greate number that hee had knowen, who (within the space of two yeares) had been furnished with *Famylyars* (Angels as hee calde them) by his masters meanes, together with the assistance of two other, who were his associates. Hee likewise tolde mee where they kept their *Randevous*, viz. in *Golding lane*, in the house of one of those Comrades (who was likewise a profest *Physition*).[75] And that at their meetings they did exercise their art, and shewde many pretty tricks unto their disciples. I further demanded of him, whether that they tooke any monye of such as came unto them, for their furnishing of them with famylyars? To which hee answered mee affirmatively that they did.

I requested him likewise to tell mee whether that his Master were not able to tell who they were, who were black (or hurting) witches, and whether hee coulde help such as were bewitched? To this hee answered that his master (uppon his knowledg) did deadly hate those kinde of people. As also that hee did much good in helping bothe men and cattell which were bewitched. I likewise entreated him to tell mee, whether his master did undertake to help men that had lost their goods, unto them agayne. This **[40]** hee confest that hee somtimes did. But in this pointe (hee sayde) hee was more close and wary, and not so free and open, as in the former.

Then: I requested him (agayne) to tell mee truely what kind of compact there was betwixt the Artists and their Angells? To this hee answered (as before) that hee coulde never com to know of any kinde of compact or covenant, that they made one with another further than this: viz. That the Angell promised to com and appeare (at all times) unto his disciple uppon the use of the *Vocabula*. But this one thing, hee tolde mee (of his owne accorde) that hee had often seen, both his master and the rest, to doe reverence unto their Angels, when they appeared unto them. The last request that I made unto him, was, that hee woulde tell mee how or by what meanes, they came to have such exact and exquisite knowledg in the judgment of urines? To this hee answered that their Angell did reveale all the secrets of the sick unto them, with each perticular circumstance thereunto appertayning. And that they required the sight or view of the urine, to shadow the secrets of their Science: heerby deluding the common people.

Dr:–: I pray you tell mee, what use made you of all this unto your self?

Phy:–: Sir: Ile tell you in breef: first (in the best manner that I coulde) I gave moste humble and harty thanks unto Almighty God, for his greate mercy unto mee, in that it had pleased his infinite goodnes, thus to discover those subtill sleyghtes of *Sathan* unto

---

[75] Golding Lane (or Golden Lane) turns north off Beech Lane.

mee; and in that hee had so graciously delyvered my soule from those his snares, wherein hee suffered many others to be caught (many whereof were knowne unto my self). Secondly, I gave my self more frequently and fervently unto prayer. And thirdly (having received this light from the servant) I adrest my self (with my best witts) to sift the Master, as often as opportunitie afforded mee any advantage thereunto.

Dr:–: In myne opinion, you did well in thus doing: But what gott you from the master?

Phy:–: Surely Sir: sufficient to make mee to leave his societie, and to loathe his Science: for by propounding Querees unto him, concerning the premises, I gradually gott out of him confession of many perticulers, which I desyred satisffaction in. Yea (one time) somthing more then I expected.**[41]** For being conferring with him aboute black witchcraft, hee tolde mee two storyes which fulfild my stomack.

Dr:–: I pray you, what were those.

History

Phy:–: Sir: first hee tolde mee that in the parrish where his lands lay, there were two black (or hurting) witches, bothe which, hee (by his art) knew to be such and for that cause desyred, to bring them bothe unto their just deserved deaths. And although there were suspicions many: and presumptions greate: yet coulde hee not get any evincing evidence against them. Whereuppon hee projected this plott aganst them, viz. so to handle matters, as to bring them to accuse one another. And er long after this; opportunity opened a way to bring his intention unto execution. For hee knowing (whether by intelligence, or otherwise) that one of those witches was gone forth on som errand, unto a yeomans house in the parrish: hee gat or procured a man of good accounte, creditt and understanding (being one of his neighbours) to walke that way with him: and as they were so walking together they mett the witch returning towards her home. The witch did humble obaysance unto him: And hee thus greeted her: Ah: you are a trim huswife indeed youle ene be hangd er long. The Witch replying sayde, Master I know you love to jeaste somtimes, but I am sure that I never deserved any such matter. But thou hast sayde hee, for thou hast bewitched to death such and such: and such an one (naming thother witch) hath accused thee for so doing: Shee replying sayde, shee lyeth like an arrant witch as shee is, for I am sure that shee did bewitch such and such, which I can justifie; well sayde the gentillman unto her I woulde wish thee to looke well unto thy self, for thou wilt speedily bee called into question for thy witchcraft, and so went on his way. And as hee went hee conferd with his neighbour, aboute the witches accusation of that other witch: praying him to remember each perticuler thereof, which hee promising to doe, they bothe forthwith went unto that other witches house: where opportunely finding her at home, this gentillman tolde her that such a woman (naming the other witch) had accused her lately unto them, to be a witch, charging her with such and such severall deeds done by her, which hee related unto her in each perticuler. This witch excused her self, (as well as shee coulde) and with greate indignation, accused the other of those and the same crymes, with the which this gentillman had formerly charged her. Heeruppon the men departe; and without any further delay, caused them bothe to be apprehended **[42]** and to be carryed aparte, unto the next Justice of the peace: who, after their severall examinations: sent them unto prison. And at the next Assises, they were bothe of them convicted, condemned, and afterwards executed.

Another storye hee tolde mee, which was as followeth. A certayne rich yeoman (who dwelt not many miles from him) had a certayne large feild, which was haunted with a wicked spirit (sent thither by a Witch) so that whatsoever cattell were put into that feilde, were smitten with som sore disease, of the which they perished, so that the owner of that land, sustayned greate loss thereby: neither remedy coulde hee gett, till at length hee hearing of this exquisite *Artist*, hee sent unto him, to enquire of him, whether that his skill, were able to afforde him remedy? This man, consulting with his Angell (as hee sayde) founde out the cause of that calamitie: with assurance of remedy, if hee shoulde be imployed in that buisines. Whereuppon hee sent back worde by the messenger, that hee coulde certaynely help all this, if in case hee woulde send for him. The Yeoman gladly embraces the offer: and without any further delay, sends forthwith for him: This *Artist* procrastinateth not the time, but went together with the messenger unto that Yeoman. They being mett; unto that grounde they goe bothe together: and surrounding the same, The *Artist* (as hee tolde mee) founde the gap, by the which the devill entred into that grounde: which, having well observed, hee likewise specially marked, that so hee mought not miss it when hee came agayne in the night. This done: they bothe returne unto the Yeomans house, where they past the time in pleasing recreation, untill the *Artist* thought it fitt to repayre unto the feilde: And thither they two went; bothe together. And in a select place, within the gap (forenamed) the *Artist* made his conjured circle. And long after it was not before the spirit came, and in that circle was captivde. Heeruppon the Spirit transforms himself into sundry shapes, to the no small wonder and amasement of the

Another: History

Yeoman: but the *Artist* encouraged him not to feare, promising to tame him in short time: which (as hee sayde) hee soone effected, bringing him to confess the combination, which was betwixt him and the witch, which sent him thither. After this, the *Artist* obliged the spirit (for ever) to relinquish that land, and not to come there agayne any more. The which uppon promise of enlargement from out that circle, hee **[43]** protested to performe. But one thing I may not forgett, which was a certayne doctrine, which (as hee tolde mee) the devill taught him, by the vertue (or rather by the vice) whereof, any man mought undoe any enemye which hee had.

Dr:–: And what mought that bee, I pray you tell us?

Phy:–: *Reverend Sir*: Ile geve you som generall notion thereof: As for the perticulers: I deeme it safest not to reveale the same, leaste thereby I shoulde shew unto men the patterne and platforme, of a moste haynous and horrible sinn. Wherefore in breef, the doctrine delyvered by the devill: was this: viz. that if hee (or any other man) woulde write *Verbatim*, a certaine psalme (which as I sayde before, I dare not name) and reade the same every morning, and then folde up the paper, and put the same into one of his shoes (but whether shoe I remember not) and so weare the same all the day betweene his foote and his shoe; and at night take it out, and reade it agayne, then folde it up, and lay it all night under the pillow, on which hee layeth his head: And the next morning, reade, folde, and weare it (all the day) as before and so agayne at night to doe with it as hee did the night before. And so constantly to keep this course, for some certayne number of dayes. That then this thing being performed: whatever partye (the person so doing) shoulde intend evill against, That party hee sayde shoulde never prosper, but decay, bothe in body and estate.

A devillish doctrine.

Dr:–: I must needs accorde with you in this; that this was a devillish doctrine indeed. For Gods worde never taught (ne yet warranteth) any such thing. Neighbour *Gregory*: what think you of this?

Greg:–: Marry zur: An ta ma pleaze your worship: chill tell you what I dee think oa tha matter: I dee think (too tell ee true) that tiz no better nor stark Witcheree. What? lurne oa tha d'vle too doo mischeife, theres a trick indeed. God bless mee, an all Crissen voke vrom tha d'vle, an all his workes.[76]

Dr:–: Tis well sayde of you: and I am right glad to heare that you conceve the pointe so right. For in such a case (as this now

[76] This sentence receives two virgules at the end (rather than Poeton's usual single virgule), perhaps for emphasis.

spoken of) to use, the worde of God: Is indeed sacrilegiously to abuse and prophane it, for that word of God is geven unto men for the ædification of their soules, and not for the hurt of their bodyes, or ruine of their estates. Wherefore so to abuse the worde of God, must needs be a worke, both impious, abhominable, and accursed.
[44] *Greg*:–: Master doctur: ee za well indeed. An too tell ee true, vor my parte cham o your verre pinnion oo a hears breadth: Oa tiz a bomminable thing indeed too lurne oa tha d'vle, too doo wonz neighbours hurt. Oa chud nut doot, no not vor all tha wealth in tha parrish, nut I.

Dr:–: Neighbour I like well of your resolution: for alas, what profitt can there be compared with the soules welfare, or what loss can be so greate as the loss of Gods favour. But to leave you a littell to your self, I must entreate Mr *Phylomathes* to goe on where hee left, and to tell us, how and in what manner hee parted with that his (so much affected) frend.

Phy:–: Sir: Ile tell you. By this history which hee last related, I plainely perceived that his skill was none other than meere diabolicall: for thus much I was confident of, that Gods worde never taught nor authorized any such art, as consists of circles, characters, crosses, charmes, spells, coniurations, *vocabulaes*, or any such like. Wherefore, (the lorde geving mee courage) I gan boldely to question the lawfullnes of his art: telling him in playne termes, that I much feared that all his shewes of sanctitie, did not proceed from sincerity, but rather, that there was some deep misterie of iniquitie in the matter.

Dr:–: How did hee take theis your speeches?

Phy:–: Surely Sir: very (seemingly) well. For hee was a man (outwardly) very well governed: and I rather think that hee was offended at himself, then angry with mee. For by that which hee thought moste certainly to have gaynde mee, hee utterly lost mee. For after the time that I had once fisht from his owne confession that hee had a familiar Angell (as hee styled him): then durst I say any thing unto him. For I spared not to tell him, that his famyliar, was none other, neither any better, than a meere devill. But this hee seemed to take somthing harshly at my hands (yet was hee much appalde therat) for hee tolde mee, that certes I had conceived much amiss. For sayde hee, the devill never instigated any one, unto that which is good: but contrariwise, still tempteth, provoketh, and alureth unto that which is evill. But the Angell (sayde hee) with whom I converse hath often exhorted mee unto this austere course of life, which you see mee lyve, and menaceth mee, that if I leave it; he then will also leave mee: Therefore it cannot be but a good Angell.

[45] *Dr*:–: I confess unto you, that hee did make a witty apologie, both for himself, as also for his familiar: how did you evince it?

Phy:–: *Reverend Sir*: (as neare as I can remember) I will relate unto you, the substance of myne answere unto him. Sir: (sayde I) admit that it be even so as you say, viz. that your familiar spirit, doe enjoyne an austere course of life unto you: Yet this is not any evincing argument whereby to prove that it is an holy Angell: For this you cannot be ignorant of, viz. that *Sathan* can transform himself into the likenes of an Angell of light: which cannot be intended to consist of any sensible shape or shew; but rather of spirituall disposition. And thus much I presume, that *Sathan* doth (often) for his owne ends, perswade his disciples to greate austeritie in outward conversation: if in the Interim; hee can but holde them captive under any one spirituall wickednes whatsoever. And further have not Idolatrous preistes and prophets, been (many times) more austere towards themselves, then the holy servants of the most high God? To instance in one onely example, (for I confess that I have not often read the scriptures, the more my shame; the greater my sinn) which is (as I remember) recorded in the eighteenth chapter of the first booke of the Kings: of the outward zeale of the prophetts of *Baal*: who cut *themselves with knyves and lancers, tyll the blood gushed out*. And as I remember theis wordes are added in the text, *as their manner was*. So that its apparant that they did not that in any furious fitt at that time, but its evident, that it was their custome so to doe, aswell at other times as then. And yet notwithstanding this greate severitie, theis were but false prophets, servants unto, yea slaves of the devill. And surely Sir, *Sathan* is sly, subtill, crafty, and cunning: and knoweth how to order all his matters and manners, in such sorte that hee thereby deludeth and deceiveth all sortes of men. To instance in your self, *Sathan* forgets not that your education, was (from your youthe) in the schoole of Christ, and founde some morrall vertues formed in you, others perchance habituated. Now you being thus furnished, and that (doubtles) with some good affections, thereto conioyned, well observed by *Sathan*, hee playnely perceived, that it woulde prejudice him in his proiect, if hee shoulde open himself unto you in any hellish hew: wherefore (God permitting) hee came disguised in the likenes of **[46]** an Angell of light: leaste otherwise hee mought (even at the first) have frighted you, and so caused in you, an utter revolt from him: Whereas now, by his seeming sanctitite, hee hath even setled you in this cursed course of life. And you are so blinded that you see not the sinns which you committ against the moste mightye and moste holy God: by abusing his moste glorious name, and worde, in the dayly practice of your charmes, characters, conjurations, spells; *vocabulaes*; and sundry the like, frequent in the exercise of your art. And then I instantly urged, and earnestly perswaded him, to consult with some Orthodox divine: and truely and fully to acquaint him with all the misteryes of his art: and to crave his councell concerning the same; and not to trust his owne hart, in a buisiness of such infinite importe, which concernd the eternall hazzard of his soule.

Greg:–: In good veth zur: I must needs ze, that you gaven good device if zo be that hee had had but zo much grace az too ha vollod your good councell. I marle much what a coud ze too tha matter?

Phy:–: Certes (honest frend) as wise as he was, yet at the first, hee was much amated,[77] and gave mee none answere at all: But after some pause: hee gan this to reason: Surely, you judg both rashly and much amiss: in that you deem my art to be diabolicall, and that you think that it is an infernall spirit, with whom I converse: but for myne owne parte, I am assuredly perswaded, that hee is a glorious Angell: and the rather to strengthen and confirme mee therein, I faythfully protest that I never founde him to have any the leaste inclination to hurt: but on the contrary very willing to discover hurting witches.

Dr:–: I pray you what did you answere unto that his Apologie?

Phy:–: I tolde him, that I much questioned, whether that hee were able to put a reall difference between the cleane and the uncleane, the pretious and the vile, neither did I think that hee had that gift from above; to discerne of spirits, and to trye the spirits whether they be of God or not? I likewise prest him with som other the like questions, as I had formerly propounded; unto that other *Artist*, from whom, God (formerly) gave mee delyverance. In close of all, I askt him whether (or not) hee founde his famylyar, forward and inclineable to drawe on others to that profession and practice? The which hee coulde not avoyde. But yet hee woulde fayne have justifyed bothe his Angell and his art, which God asisting mee I still beate him from; so as in fine hee desperately **[47]** brast[78] forthe and sayde: have I not often preached unto thee; and doest thou now preach unto mee? I pray thee talke no more to mee of this matter. For thou and I each day ask vengance agaynst our selves; and wee are none other then damned creatures. And uppon theis wordes

[77] Dismayed, overwhelmed, confounded.

[78] According to the *OED* this is a northern dialect form of "burst."

hee departed from mee, and from thenceforth, hee never woulde admitt any conference with mee.

Dr:–: The more happy you: but the more unhapppy hee.

Greg:–: Ye ze verry true indeed (Mr doctur). A must needs bee unhappy indeed, that dee think a shall bee damnd; an that ha no hope too bee saved.

Dr:–: Tis right so neighbour, but suffer mee (I pray you) to ask Mr *Phylomathes*, another question or two.

Greg:–: Is with all my hart zur.

Dr:–: Mr *Phylomathes*, I pray you tell mee, coulde you never com unto the certayne knowledg of the compact which is made twixt *Sathan* and those *Sorcerers*?

Phy:–: Surely, Sir: at the first (for ought that ever I coulde learne) they doe not. But in proces of time, the devill drawes them in by degrees. For if hee shoulde at the first, appeare unto them, such an one as hee is: few there are of theis, but that they woulde fly from him. Wherefore, that sly and subtill Serpent, seems (for a tyme) contented; with some reverence and worship, by them, to be performed to him, with their sacrilegious prophanations of the moste sacred name and worde of God: And to strengthen and confirme them therein: hee coming masqued under a vayle of sanctitie, will press them not onely unto some negative vertues, as not to sweare, not to be drunk, and the like. But hee will also excite them unto some affirmative holy dueties: as to make an outwarde profession of religion, to repayre to the church, to heare sermons, to receive the Sacraments, yea to talke and confer of the word of God: Yea further heele perswade them to performe som seeming charitable acts: As freely (in some cases) to geve counsell and advice, yea to administer help unto the poore, and unto such as are in distress: for Sathan is Gods Ape, desyring (in all things) to imitate him. Whence it cometh to pass, that sundry wise and learned men (after the flesh) have been (in all ages) seduced by *Sathan*, who have thought themselves (by theis their courses) to be even rapt up into heaven: when alas (poore soules) they were (even headlong) hurryed unto hell.

Dr:–: I conceive theis things, which you have spoken, to be noe less then **[48]** truthe. But how comes it to pass that the devill will be observant unto theis without some greater salarie: to witt the gayning of their soules?

Phy:–: *Reverend Sir*: it pleaseth you to ask this question of mee, rather to try how I can answere it, then that you need any solution therein. But to answere (according to my weaknes) the devill is like an affected *Gamester*, who will (according to the proverb) play small game, rather than hee will sit out.

Dr:–: Express your self more fully.

Phy:–: *Sir*: my meaning (in playne termes) is this: That *Sly Serpent*, well observeth the severall disposition, of each perticular man, warily weighing his affections, and carefully considereth how hee standeth (more or less) adicted to religion. And so accordingly addresseth himself to each attempt. To instance: If hee finde a man (in any sorte) to be piously adicted: then, to such an one heele shew himself in likenes of a Saint, exhorting them to an austere lyfe, and dehorting them from the common vices of the times; contenting himself for the time, that they use the vocabula: and that they exercise themselves in the freqent use of some supersticious prayers: then heele teach them charmes and spells: and so gradually draw them on, unto an high measure of sinning against God. And to theis hee is is exceedingly observant, to afforde them all the delight and content that hee can invent or devise, untill that hee hath fastened their affections unto a love and liking of this pestilent practice. But then heel fayle, either to direct or asist them, in those thinges, which they moste desyre to know or doe, unles that then they will enter into covenant, and make compact with him.

Sathans policies to get his servants into a sure compact with him.

Greg:–: But pray tell mee won thing zur: cante the geen over, whon the lust?

Phy:–: No surely, unles that God of his infinite mercye vouchsafe to pluck them out of the snare of the devill: which of his speciall grace and favor hee somtimes doth, for the magnifying of his mercy, and the gloryfying of his grace and goodnes. But this is but seldom seen. For it is just with God, to geve such over into the handes of Sathan, (as doe forsake the guidance of his worde, and run a whooring after wicked inventions) whom when *Sathan* hath thus caught, hee still laboures, by all meanes possible, to keep them in captivitie. So that if any of those (who have once entered so far into that path of perdition) shall but offer to revolt and goe back: Loe then their fayre Angell will soone unmask himselfe, and shew himselfe to bee such an one as (in truthe) hee is: to witt a foule feend. Then will hee let such understand that all **[49]** those former ceremonies which they have used, were none other then hiddeous and horrible sinnes: in regarde whereof hee will tell them that its in vayne for them to think of a revolt, for they are his already, and in that respect, it can be no further prejudice unto them to enter covenant with him. The which if they will accept, that then hee (for his parte) will moste faythfully performe all such articles, conditions, and covenants, as they shall agree uppon. And thus first by flattery and fraude hee getts them into the snare, and after that keeps them captive by feare or force: otherwise if hee can, heele dryve them to despayre, and so draw them to some desperate end.

Greg:–: Now God bless mee, an keep mee vrom tha d'vle, an all his workes: It zeems that a is peslance zuttell: But vor my parte cham rezolvd (zo cham) nere too ha enny thing too doo wene, nor with enny won that belongs toon, zo neare az can, by tha grace a God.

Dr:–: Tis well sayde, and well resolved of you, and I pray God to keep you in that minde still. But Mr *Phylomathes* tell mee, what are the covenants that pass between them, if Sathan so prevayle?

Phy:–: As I have been informed, the devill requires of some that they become wholely his, that is to geve themselves unto him, bothe bodye and soule. And theis are such, as either hee findes to be desperately minded alreardye, or else drawne to be such by his devellish devices. Of others (at first) hee requires worship and service, with the which, for a time, hee seems to be contented. But yet watcheth hee continually all opportunities, to make them wholly his.

Dr:–: And what doth the devill (on his parte) promise unto such?

Phy:–: Surely Sir: (as I have heard) to appeare unto them, when they shall use the wordes of their vocabula. To reveale unto them, what they desyre to know. To doe for them whatever is in his power to performe. To instance in some perticulars. To reveale (aforehand) unto healing witches, who shall com unto them: as also from whom, and for what. And uppon the presentation of an urine: to make knowne unto them, the full state of a sick person, with the Antecedent and primitive causes of their greefs, together with the severall circumstances, concommitances, accidents, and Symptomes thereof. And this hee doth to some, by speaking in their eare: before some heel seemingly disect the body of the **[50]** sick pointing unto every parte thats ill affected, distempered, or diseased. Unto other some, heel present a fayre printed table in the Ayre, which shalbe onely seen of the *Artist*: wherein he may reade whatever hee desyreth to know. And so to be ready furnished with prompt answeres: unto whatever shall be propounded unto him. Hence such as these, reape such rare creditt from the common people. And all theis misteryes of that their art were revealed unto mee, by one *Woodrofe* a *Taylor*, a *Lyncolnshyre* man, who had been a servant unto one of those famous *Sorcerers* formerly spoken of: who (likewise himself) was new entred into that filthy fraternitie.

How they com to be so skilfull in urines.

Hee further tolde mee that (if they require it) their Angell will disclose and discover unto them, such as are black (or hurting) witches: with their dwelling places: In what place they keep they famylyars: As also where, or in what parte of the witches body, the devill hath markt him or her. Now in regarde of this their superexcelling science, in waters, and discovering of witchcraft, they are held, reputed, and taken to bee, the meer Monopolists of Art: As for such as deale by lawfull and lawdable art, those are for the moste parte, neglected and contemned.

Dr:–: Sir: as I remember, you formerly sayde that those kinde of people, are meanely stored with medicines: How comes it then to pass, that they cure such varyetie of maladyes?

Phy:–: Sir: on their medicines they relye not at all: (as hath been confest unto mee by some of their owne *sect*). They geve, or appoint some things onely to vayle their villanyes withall. They principally repose their confidence (for the cure) in their famyliar.

Dr:–: But can the devill effect any cure immediately, or without meanes, think you?

Phy:–: No certes (in my judgement) hee cannot. But this I am perswaded of; that the devill (God permitting) is able to extract, the Quintessance, vertue, life, or spirit (terme it how you please) out of any (either) vegetall, or minerall, and so convay the same into the bodyes either of men or beastes: and that far more accurately, then can be performed, by any ordinary Artist, be hee never so exquisite.[79]

How or by what meanes the devill effects cures.

Dr:–: It seems that you are perswaded, that *Sathan* is well acquainted with the secrets of nature: and that hee is no less then an *Arch Alchymist.*[80]

[51] *Phy*:–: I am no less perswaded indeed.

---

[79] In this context, careful, skilful, accomplished; see *OED* entry at 2a and 4.

[80] Satan's extensive knowledge of nature and natural processes was a demonological commonplace. Though fallen, he was still angelic in nature, not to mention of exceedingly great age, and he retained a degree of knowledge and understanding which far surpassed that of humans. Much magic and other occult activity (including alchemy) relied—according to its opponents—on the Devil's assistance in this regard. See Clark, *Thinking With Demons*, chap. 11. Poeton seems to be using the term "alchemist" fairly broadly here, including within it practitioners of natural magic and occult healing more generally.

Dr:–: What is your opinion, concerning the weapon salve: together with the cures thereby effected?[81]

Cure by the weapon salve.

Phy:–: *Sir*: I dare not to judg it, because judgment appertaynes not unto mee. But under correction, of those who are wise, learned, and judicious: Ile freely delyver my poore opinion: which is: I think that the devill hath a finger, if not a hand therein.

Dr:–: What reasons have you so to think?

Phy:–: Sir: myne opinion ariseth from reason, otherwise it shoulde have no habitation in my hart. The first reason therefore moving mee so to think, is, because that the first Author thereof, was a very Witch.

Dr:–: What authoritie have you for that?

Phy:–: Mr *Bernard*:[82] (in his *Guide to Grand Iury men*: *booke* 2. *ch*. 7. *page* 122.) quotes *Keckerman*,[83] for his authoritie in this pointe, who sayth that one *Anselmus*[84] was the Author thereof: who was a very Witch. And Mr *Foster*[85] in *his booke called A spunge to wipe of the weapon salve*, sayes that one *Paracelsus*[86] was the *Author* thereof: whom hee likewise affirmeth to be a very witch.

---

[81] The weapon-salve was a form of sympathetic magic which involved anointing the bloodstained weapon as a method of treating the wound it had caused. See introduction and following notes.

[82] Richard Bernard, author of *A Gvide To Grand-Ivry Men* (1627). Poeton uses the second edition of 1629 (reissued 1630).

[83] Bartholomäus Keckermann (c. 1571–1608/9) was a German Calvinist theologian. Foster cites Keckermann's *Systema Physicvm* (Hanau: William Anthony, 1612) for discussion of the weapon-salve.

[84] Anselm of Parma (1386–1440), scientist and author of a work on magic, *De magia disciplina*. Opinion was divided in the period as to whether he was a sorcerer or a natural philosopher. A recent defence by Gabriel Naudé had appeared in 1625; see the English translation, *The History of Magick*, trans. John Davies (London: John Streater, 1657), 175.

[85] William Foster, author of *Hoplocrismaspongvs: Or, A Sponge to wipe away the Weapon-Salve* (1631). Foster, a Buckinghamshire clergyman, argued that the weapon-salve was diabolical in nature, tantamount to witchcraft. He was arguing in particular against Robert Fludd (see below).

[86] Paracelsus (1493–1541) was a notorious German physician, alchemist, and occultist. He rejected much of classical medical theory and practice, insisting on the value of observations of nature. His work was very influential across Europe, and he had a large following in England but, as this passage makes clear, there were many who considered his work diabolical. The invention of the weapon-salve was often erroneously ascribed to him. Foster does so (*A Sponge*, 13–15), although he notes with Poeton and Bernard that Keckermann laid it at the door of Anselm of Parma. Foster writes of the weapon-salve:

Dr:–: But coulde there be two severall Authors of one and the same salve?

Phy:–: There are, (as I have been credibly informed) two (if not more) severall receipts thereof: so that there may be two Authors likewise, and bothe of them Witches.

Dr:–: You say well therein. But, alow those to be witches, and that they were taught to make the medicine, by the devill: yet now you see that sundry honest, weldisposed, conscionable *Christians*, make use thereof, and effect marvelous cures thereby. I hope that you doe not conceite such men to be Witches?

Phy:–: Sir: I neither doe, nor dare say that such are witches: and yet notwithstanding, there may be witchcraft in the matter.

Dr:–: As how I pray you?

Phy:–: By an implicite compact.

Dr:–: Express your self more fully.

Phy:–: I conceive that the case in this pointe, is not much unlike a contract **[52]** or covenant made betweene, the Lessour and the Lessee, wherein the Lessour covenanteth with the Lessee, his executors &c. that if hee the sayde Lessee, his executors &c. shall observe, fulfill, keep, and doe, such and such things, that then they shall enjoy, such and such priveledges, and prerogatives. I apply it thus. I conceve that *Sathan*, was the prime Author of this supernaturall Art:[87] and that hee imparted the same, unto some of his disciples, (who were in compact or covenant with him): with an entayle, of that curing prærogative, unto their disciples, and unto the disciples of their disciples, (in perpetuitie) uppon condition, that

Quoad homines.

> Now then *Paracelsus* being a Witch, and this experiment being placed amongst his Diabolicall and magicall conclusions, it cannot chooce but be Witchcraft, and come from the grand master of Witches the Diuell, if *Paracelsus* were (as most repute him) the Author and Founder of it. Neither can it be better, if *Anselmus* were the Authour of it, as *Keckerman* reports. For, saith the same *Keckerman*, this *Anselmus* (howsoever he is by some now esteemed) was a noted Magician whilst hee lived.
>
> Foster, *A Sponge*, 15.

According to Lauren Kassell, the weapon-salve was in fact first promoted in a pseudo-Paracelsian work of 1570, and then more widely publicised in 1589 by Giovanni Battista Della Porta; "Magic, Alchemy and the Medical Economy," in Jenner, Mark S. R. and Wallis, Patrick, eds., *Medicine and the Market in England and Its Colonies, c. 1450–c. 1850* (Basingstoke: Palgrave Macmillan, 2007), 91–92.

[87] *Quoad homines*: in respect of men. This note is underlined, as is "supernaturall Art" in the body text, in what looks this time like Poeton's ink.

they making and ordering that medicine: according to his rules præscribed, that then hee woulde effect the cure. But unto all theis you must conceve, that credence must be conjoyned: otherwise I question not, but that the cure will fayle, and all their worke be frustrate.

And for myne owne parte, I durst engage all that meane estate that I possess, uppon it, that lett any one of those Opperators, delyver into my hands the weapon, and the medicine, together with all rules for the ordering of bothe: and that though I shoulde never swerve from prescription in the performance of each thing appointed: that yet thereby there shoulde not be any cure effected. And my grounde for this myne opinion is, that I cannot fynde any the leaste foundation for fayth to be built uppon; my meaning (in sum) is that there is not any worde of God to warrant such a course as this; for the effecting of such a cure.

Dr:–: I cannot but approve that which you have spoken, to be very probeable: but yet there is a learned doctor of *Physick* who hath written a tract in defence thereof. Have you not seen it? Its called the squeasing of *Parson Fosters spunge.*[88]

Phy:–: Yes *Sir*: I have bothe seen and read it.

Dr:–: And what say you of it?

Phy:–: I must needs confes, that its a very learned worke, and hee is a noble gentillman that wrote it. But if I remember aright, uppon the close of the cure: hee brings in the *Spirit* of the Ayre, to carry the *Balsam* of the effused blood, together with the Quintessence of the salve from the weapon to the wounde. Now if that learned gentillman meane that spirit that ruleth in the ayre, Ile soone seale to that sentence.[89]

[53] *Dr*:–: You doe well to geve that doctor his due: And as for that worke of his, I freely say of it, that it is bothe learned and laborious. As for your collection and close: I say no more of it than thus: though it be curt: yet may it pass for currant. But now lets leave this

[88] Robert Fludd, *Doctor Flvdds Answer unto M. Foster Or, The Sqvesing Of Parson Fosters Sponge, ordained by him for the wiping away of the Weapon-Salve* (1631). This tract was, as the title suggests, a response to Foster's tract, in defence of the weapon-salve. Fludd argues for the natural efficacy of the cure. He was a respected member of the Royal College of Physicians, and his support for the belief shows that it was not an idea from the outer margins of early modern culture; this is presumably why Poeton is unwilling to criticise him too fiercely.

[89] The reference is perhaps to page 45 in Fludd. The "spirit that ruleth in the ayre" is of course Satan; see Ephesians 2:2.

matter as twere in the midst: and pass on unto some other pointe. I pray you tell mee your opinion concerning the boy of Godlyman, that Fidlers seventh Sonn; surnamed (by some) the yong prophet of Godlyman: I have heard that there is much resorte unto him, and that greate cures have been done by him.[90]

The yong prophet, of Godlyman.

Phy:–: Certes *Sir*: I never saw him (that I know of) but I have heard as much of him, as you have now spoken.

Dr:–: But what think you of his actions, be they lawfull or not?

Phy:–: *Reverend Sir*: your self is better able to judg of them, than I am: in respect of your constant conversing in the sacred scriptures: you can tell whether or not, that the Almighty hath entayled the gift of healing, uppon a seventh sonn, successively succeeding one another, from the self same parents.

Dr:–: That there is any promise made to such a person, to such a purpose, is more then ever I saw, read, or heard: But in what manner doth hee effect the cures which hee doth?

Phy:–: *Sir*: therein I can speake none otherwise, than uppon others reportes: neither did I ever talke with any that had been his patient, save one onely woman of *Kirdford*:[91] and as shee tolde me, when as shee first went unto him, shee was in a very ill case, with an ulcer in her face, neare unto her left eye; with sundry painfull swellings aboute that side of her face, head and neck. The which sore and swellings hee did onely stroke with his hand, at sundry times, and so shee was recovered. Then I demanded of her whether hee did not use any wordes, in the performance of the cure? To the which shee answered that hee did speake some thinges secretly to him self, but what it was that hee sayde, shee knew not. Now I desyre to know of you what you think of theis things?

Dr:–: *Sir*: Ile freely declare unto you, my minde concerning theis matters. Wherefore in the curing of all diseases, there ought meanes to be used, neither ought wee to expect miracles now in theis dayes, in the **[54]** which the gospell is now confirmed and setled among us. Now seeing that it is so, that all diseases (which admit cure) are cured either by meanes naturall, or by power supernaturall: If by meanes naturall, then are such as are learned,

---

[90] Godlyman is Godalming in Surrey, around 30 miles due north of Petworth. This boy, for whom Poeton is apparently the only source, is a "stroker," one who heals by touch. Belief in this power was relatively common during the period, and such figures were often seventh sons. See introduction.

[91] Kirdford is a village in West Sussex, around four miles northeast of Petworth. Earlier in the text it is given in reverse as Drofdrik.

judicious, experienced, to be sought unto: to be used and imployed, in and aboute the effecting of cures: others (not so quallyfyed) to be refused. On the other side, if cures be effected by supernaturall power: either it must be from God who is able to doe all things, by the worde of his power; Or else from *Sathan* (that greate Inspector of nature) by his cuning extracting, and subtill applying of the vertues, or vertuall spirits, of medicinable creatures: unto diseased persons. Now to speake properly, theis kind of cures thus effected, by *Sathans* art and industrye, cannot (in truthe of divinitie), be justly termed supernaturall, because that Sathan himself is a creature natured, bounded, limited, beyond which hee cannot (in any sorte) pass. And therefore wee abusively call *Sathans* Sly and subtill workings, by the name of miracles, which to worke is only proper and peculiar unto Almighty God, who onely and alone doth wonderfull things. So that all those secret subtill workings of *Sathan*, in, by, and with the creatures, may not unfitly be termed strange, or marvelous, but truely miraculous they are not, ne can (in any sorte) be. For so to speake, is to rob God of his glory. Wherefore to proceed, in this pointe in hand. Wee humbly and reverently acknowledg: that the Lord created all things of nothing: and that hee alone ruleth and reigneth over all: doing whatsoever pleaseth him, whether in heaven, earth, seas, or else where: and that hee ordereth all thinges according to the purpose of his owne will: which will of his wee beleeve and acknowledg to be, the rule of all righteousness. So that whatsoever it be, that is not leveled according to the rightnes of that moste sacred will of God, how seeming strayght or equall soever it may seem to be in the eyes of men: yet if once it be brought to that rule, and layde to that levell, its crookednes and curvitie,[92] will right soone be seen, of such as are inlightned from above. Now to come to som use of what hath been sayde, and to apply these things to our present purpose: Not to cite agayne that miracle of *Myracles*; the Creation: ne yet to speake of his inverting the course **[55]** of nature: As in dividing the red Sea, causing the waters to stand on an heape &c. As also (in the dayes of *Joshua*) in stopping the Sun of his course, and causing him to stand still (in the midst of heaven) and not to hasten to goe downe, by the space of a whole day,[93] with many the like miracles of his moste marvelous power: of the which wee may reade in sundry places of sacred writt. But to desist from theis: weele now consider such miracles as God hath wrought by

[92] Poeton originally wrote "pervisitie" but corrected it to "curvitie," perhaps to remove a sense of moral judgement from the term?

[93] Joshua 10:13.

his servants, concerning the cure of bodily diseases and infirmities: wherein for method and memory sake, lets observe first what sortes of people, God hath ever used, in the effecting of those his marvelous workes in the curing of bodily infirmities &c. Secondly weele examine the meanes whereby. And lastly weele paralel, our yong *Godlyman Prophet* with those former instruments, by whom God wrought those greate workes of his mercy uppon the afflicted and distressed. Wherefore to begin with *Elijah*: and consider who hee was: what hee did: and how, or by what meanes, hee did it? *1 Kings 17. 1.*
First who hee was? *Hee* was an holy prophett of the *Lord*: A type of *Matthew 11. 10. 14.*
the holy *Baptist*: one who together with *Moses*, appeared unto, and conferred with our blessed *Saviour* in the mount: A man zealous *Matthew 17. 3.*
for the *Lord of hosts*. This holy prophett (through the power of God) *1 Kings 19. 10.*
wrought a greate miracle, uppon the widdowes sonn of *Zarephath*, whom hee raysed from death to life: But the manner how hee did it, is likewise to be considered. For first its written that hee cryed unto the lorde: hee contented not himself with *lip labour*, to patter over a *pater noster*, or to mumble up an *Ave Mary*, but hee prayde with the understanding: in the spirit, with fayth, with fervencye with perseverance: untill the lord heard him and raysed the childe from death to life. In like manner, *Elysha* (*another* holy prophet of *1 Kings 17. 20. 21. 22.*
the Lord) raysed to life, the sonn of the *Shunanite*: which hee likewise did by faythfull and fervent prayer. And by the power of the *2 Kings 4.*
worde of the lorde (in the mouth of that holy *Elysha*) was *Naaman* the *Sirian* clensed from his leprosye, by washing himself seven tymes in Jordan. Lets now pass from the holy Prophets: and com *2 Kings 5.*
to the bessed Apostles, and faythfull disciples of our sweet Saviour the Lord Jesus. Let us looke on (and consider) their mission: their comission; their priveledges: with the effects and success of each of those. Those blessed Apostles (before our Saviours suffrings) were sent unto the Jewes. *Matthew* 10. 6. But after our Saviours suf fringes, they were sent unto all nations. *Matthew* 28. 19. *Mark* 16. 15. Their comission was to preach, and to say *The kingdome of heaven is at hand*. Their priviledges were: *to heale the sick, to clense* **[56]** the Lepers, to rayse the dead, and to cast out devills. Now a worde or two of their success in their proceedings. And first: In the dayes that our Saviour lyved (in the flesh) uppon the earth, hee sent forth Seventie other disciples (besides his Apostles) by two and two into every *City* and place whether hee himself woulde com. And unto *Luke 10.*
theis hee gave comission, as to the former, and endowed them with equall priveledges. As may appeare by the sequell. For those disciples returned rejoycing that the devills were subject unto them, through the name of *Christ*. Agayne: after the passion, resurrection,

and ascention of our blessed Saviour: his holy Apostles, and disciples wrought many miracles; which are recorded by St *Luke* in the holy *Acts of* the *Apostles*, in sundry and severall chapters of that holy booke. But now observe (I beseech you) that all those who wrought myracles either under the law, or under the gospell, they were men (not boyes or children), preachers of the worde of God; Ambassadors from God, unto his people, to shew and declare unto them the way of salvation. They were such as were filled with the holy *Ghost*, and furnished with all heavenly graces: necessary for the discharge of that their high and holy calling. But alas, this our yong Prophet, hath not so much as one worde out of Gods booke, to warrant either his profession or practice: Let him shew a warrant for what hee doth, for what hee sayth: and then (for myne owne parte) Ile seale up my lippes, and say nothing of him. But some *Apologize* for him and say that what hee doth, hee was instigated, and encouraged thereunto, by a doctor of *Physick*, a greate travayler, who revealed unto his parents the first light of this sublunarye secret. But where is his warrant? let him shew it of Gods word, and then Ile subscribe thereto. But in case that hee tell us of traditions: then let him prove them to be Apostolicall, And then Ile approve, that so proved. But if neither of these can be produced: then must I rest resolved that this yong prophett, is none other then a meere Impostor. And safely may I say: that all is not gould which glystereth.

Greg:–: Well vare your good hart Master doctur: my thinks that you ha zed zommwhat too tha buisines indeed: In my zimple pinnion you ha zet a shrode spoake ins cart, zo you ha: vor too tell ee true an if a ha noe warrant vrom God, vor what a dee doo, I cante zee **[57]** howt shud bee good. Vor myne none parte: chill nere goe toon, while I dee leeve, zo I wonte: And (beecause ee ar my vrends) too tell ee my minde vreely: Cham much a veard tha tha d'vle hath zum hond in tha buzines: what think you ote Mr *Phymolathes*?

Phy:–: I confess that there are some shrewd presumptions, which may geve occasion so to think: for no longer agoe then yesterday, it was tolde mee by one (whom I dare to creditt) that heard from som of his patients; that hee enjoyneth them to be fasting when they com unto him, to be touched by him, as also that hee contineweth fasting untill that hee hath finished his mornings task or travell. Now if it be so, then is it superstition at the best, if I conceve aright: and mee thinks that it mindeth towards some of the wayes of white witchcraft.

Dr:–: Sir: I think, that in speaking of that which you now have sayde, you have no way swarved from the right: And to confirme what you have spoken, Ile strengthen your opinion with some few reasons. And first I reason thus. *Hee* who effecteth cures, without naturall meanes; must needs have som supernaturall help.

But our young *Prophet of Godlyman* effecteth cures, without naturall meanes. *Ergo*: our yong *Prophet* must have som supernaturall help.[94]

Agayne.

Hee who effecteth cures in the name of God: is able to shew warrant for the same, from out the worde of God.

But our yong *Prophet*, cannot shew warrant for what hee doth, from out the word of God. *Ergo*. Our yong *Prophet* doth not effect cures in the name of God. Agayne.

Hee who effecteth cures: neither by meanes naturall: ne yet by divine asistance: must necessarily doe it by the help of the devill.

But our yong *Prophet* effects his cures: neither by meanes naturall: ne yet by divine asistance. *Ergo*. Our yong *Prophet* must necessarily doe it by the help of the devill. *Quoad homines.*

Greg:–: Ee ze well master doctur: An vor myne owne part, I cham nut able too justifie that a dee doo. But it mee thinks that zitch a yong lad as hee iz, shud nut bee acquainted with tha d'vle. Alas vorn poore childe, I donte think that hee dee think enny hurt **[58]** in what a dee doo: Shure that doctur waz much too blame, that did zetten on at vurst: zo a waz.

Dr:–: I think so to: But yet notwithstanding: hee ought to be admonished, and not to be let alone in this unwarrantable course. For suppose that hee hath not as yet made any covenant, or contract with Sathan: yet (for mine owne parte) I cannot see, how that that which hee doth shoulde in any sorte be lawfull, unless it can be warranted by the worde of God. And that it is not warranted by that worde I have formerly shewne. Now: were hee capeable of reason to discerne of naturall operations, then doubtles, hee woulde (even as man) refuse it. But were hee grounded in religion, and il luminated from on high, then (as a Christian) hee woulde utterly abhor it. But being both yong and ignorant, his case is much to be pittied: and hee ought (in charitie) to be plucked from out the snare of the devill.

Greg:–: But (master doctur) let mee make zo bolde wee, az to ax ee won question.

Dr:–: Speake freely on.

[94] In this and the preceding paragraph, "supernatuall help" is underlined, as is the marginal note, in what looks like Poeton's ink.

Greg:–: An if I mistook nut, I hurd you ze, that you thought, that hee waz not it in enny covenant with tha d'vle: wooll tha d'vle doo enny thing vor them that bente in covenant wene?

Dr:–: Yes undoubtedly hee both will and often doth, asist such, as attempt the use of unlawfull meanes. For when they will doe such things, which neither, in themselves: ne yet by any warrant from Gods worde, have power to effect that, which they endevour to bring to pass thereby. Then (doubtles) the devill will industruously endevour, to accomplish what they desyre, that by his so doing, hee may even devote them to the prosccution of those unwarrantable practises: Implicitely, becoming thereby the devills disciples: for so long as any walketh in his wayes; hee will accomodate them, in what they desyre, to the utmost of his abillities.

Greg:–: But pray zur, how may they bee zed too bee tha d'vles diziples, whan the nere goe toon, to lurne enny thing oane?

Dr:–: I answere you neighbour: such, bothe may be and are, the mediate disciples of the devill, though (in truthe) they immediately learne not any thing from him. For if they learne and practice, those thinges of the which the devill was the first inventor: I then see nothing to the **[59]** contrary, but that they may justly be denominated his disciples. For hee who is not against Sathan, is with him, and cannot lightly speake evill of him, that is of his working power: because of that implicite league that they have with him: as also in regarde of that outwarde commodity that doth accrue unto them by that their pernicious practice. This pointe may easily be proved, by the rule of contraryes: For as wee may reade *Mark* 9. *ver.* 38. 39. 40. where St *John* spake unto our Saviour, saying, *Master, wee saw one casting out devils in thy name, and hee followed not us, and wee forbade him, because he followed not us. But Jesus said, forbid him not, for there is no man, which shall doe a myracle in my name, that can lightly speake evill of mee. For he that is not against us, is on our part.*

Greg:–: Master doctur: ee ha zed verry well my thinks, An I cante tell well how theale bee able too answert. But won thing I dee marle at, whuch iz this. Theck zame *Proffet* doant help all that goe toone, what shud bee tha reazon o that, think you?

Dr:–: The reason thereof is not hard to be founde out. Which I conceve to be this. Wee are to understand that the devills cannot doe any thing more then God permitts them to doe. Now it pleaseth the Lord sometimes to suffer them to worke marvelous things in the eyes of unregenerate men: to that end that the sonns of men may be tryed whether or no that they have true and sounde knowledg of the word, wayes, and workes of the Lord. And whether they be able to put a reall difference between the cleane and the uncleane; the precious and the vile. And further, if *God* shoulde permit *Sathan* to heale and help all such as seek unto his disciples; then woulde the greater number of men, run a whooring after such, and wholely neglect, those men and meanes, which God hath sett aparte to serve his divine providence, for the health and help of his afflicted ones. And if God shoulde not suffer *Sathan* to effect som cures, where then were the cognisance of such as truely feare God to be founde out, or how mought those (in this pointe) be distinguished from the impious and prophane people of the worlde?

Greg:–: Master doctur: I dee thank ee with all my hart, vor your groate paynes and gentellnes: vor ee ha vully desolved mee in ery thing that avore chwaz ingrant of, wherevore Ile expounde no moore questions untee at this tyme. But ene now take my leave oye.

Dr:–: My good neighbour: The peace of God be allwayes with you.

Finis.

Appendix

The list beginning on page 35 is a slightly modified version of a list given by Richard Bernard in his *A Gvide To Grand-Ivry Men* (1627). Compare Bernard's list:

The good Witches (vntruely so called) may be sundry wayes knowne.

I. From the *qualitie* of the party, one commonly very ignorant of religion, an oberuer of times, of good & bad dayes, of good and bad lucke, very superstitious in many things, not induring willingly such as feare God, and such as delight in his Word. They are also fantastically proud, as *Simon Magus* was, who boasted much of himselfe, as these doe of their gift and power; as those in Spaine, which call themselues *Salutadorres*.

II. By his or her vnwillingnesse to conferre, either with godly and learned Diuines, of their Faith & good prayers, by which they professe to do such cures, or with godly and learned Physicians, about such medicines as they prescribe to procure health: both which they auoid, lest their works of darknesse should come to light, and they be discouered to bee Witches.

III. By their priuate and secret whisperings, mumblings and mutterings with a low voice, as was the manner of Witches to doe in old time, Isa. 8.19. & 29.4.

IV. By professing to bee able to helpe such as bee bewitched and forespoken: for the supernaturall worke of the diuell, as in case of bewitching, cannot be cured (as learned men affirme) by any natural meanes: this Witches haue confessed also, and therefore must be by a league betweene the Diuel and the Witch.

V. By the meanes which they doe vse to helpe such as come to them for helpe: as

By onely touching the party: *Bodinus* giueth instances, who thus cured the Ague & Toothach. 2. By saying certaine prayers, as *Anne Baker* did, and *Ioane Willimot*: which be Popish set prayers many of them; as so many Creeds, Aue-Maries and Pater-nosters, as a Witch confessed to me. 3. By Charmes and Spels, absurd, barbarous and ridiculous forms of words, and such like meanes, which haue no power from naturall working, nor from the ordinance of God, and therefore must needs be from the Diuell.

VI. By the *remedies* which these prescribe unto others to doe, to haue helpe, as one or two medicines for all diseases, impossible in nature to bee auaileable in so great varietie, and therefore do no good, and are prescribed onely to couer their diabolicall practice and Witchery. So to prescribe medicines made of such things, as are abhorring to nature, of which *Bodin* maketh mention. To prescribe Charmes, popish prayers, popish superstitions, and very Witcheries themselues, as to hang Amulets about the necke, and certaine pieces of holy Scripture, to goe and scratch the suspected, to burne some of his or her haire, or some part of the beast bewitched, to pricke a needle or bodkin vnder the stoole where the Witch sitteth, to make a Witch-cake of Bakers meale, and the bewitched parties Vrine: see for this and some others the like vanities, in Master *Roberts* practices, vnbefitting reasonable men, and sober Christians.

VII. By their foreknowledge to tell who those be that come to them, why, and for whom they come. Thus could the Witch of *Endor* tell, that he that came disguised, was *Saul.* Thus could hee that made the Witchcake, tel the party which came to him to helpe his wife, of whom Master *Roberts* doth write. That such are Witches, *Bodinus* bringeth instances out of Flanders, Portugall, France. To tel also who are bewitched, and how, and who are Witches, and where their marke is; these be Witches: for all these things they know by their spirit, as *Ioane Willimot* the Leicestershire Witch did confesse; part hereof in her first, & part in her second examination, before seuerall Iustices. For this foreknowledge Physicians haue not by their Art, neither haue these ignorant persons this by diuine inspiration, and therefore by compact with the Diuell.

VIII. By shewing the suspected in a Glasse, as hee that made the Witchcake did, before mentioned, who shewed the Witch *Mary Smith* in a Glasse. *Fernelius* speaketh of such a Witch, whom he, as himselfe saith, saw. This is an vndoubted marke of a Witch, as one Master *Edmunds* of Cambridge told me, who was one that for a time professed to helpe men to goods or money stolne, who was once by the heads of the Vniuersitie questioned, as he confessed to mee, when hee had better learned Christ, and giuen ouer his practice that way. He told mee two things (besides many others, in a whole afternoones discourse at *Castlehiningham* in Essex) neuer to bee forgotten. 1. That by his Art he could find out him that stole from another, but not for himselfe. 2. That the ground of this Art was not so certaine, but that hee might mistake, and so peraduenture accuse an honest man, in stead of the offender, and therefore gaue it ouer, albeit he said hee might haue made two hundred pound *per annum* of his skill.

IX. By paines and like torment comming vpon this good Witch, which is vpon the bewitched. Conference I had once with a suspected healing Witch, a man miserable poore, and of an horrid countenance, of whom I asking how hee knew a man or beast to be bewitched, hee told mee by two things. *First*, by his trouble in saying his prayers for the bewitched, which then he could hardly remember, and much adoe he had to make an end of them; which prayers were so many Creeds, so many Aue-Maries, so many Pater nosters. *Secondly*, by the paine which would seaze on himselfe as soone as he began his prayers, the very same which was vpon the bewitched. This skill hee learned of a woman, which taught him a secret, but what that ground of this Witchcraft was, that could I by no meanes procure him to reueale. Some know who are bewitched, as before I shewed, by their spirit, & some by some Witchery means, of which *Bodinus* maketh mention, and of many vaine people yet put in practice, when they suspect a party; for which they deserued to be punished, if they had their desert.

X. Lastly, by requiring Faith of such as come unto them: Physicians expect it not, neither dare any truely fearing God, rob thus God of his honour (who curseth such as trust in man) and yet these VVitches professe, that they cannot heale such as doe not beleeue in them. This *Bodinus* sheweth by examples three or foure, whereof one *Healer* came to a Bishop, and willed him to trust in him to cure him, and this was in the hearing of *Bodinus* himselfe, there in the Chamber, and one Doctor *Faber*, a learned Physician. Thus may these, falsely so named good VVitches, be discouered.

A Gvide To Grand-Ivry Men, chap. 8, 132–40.

Note in particular that Poeton adds a final entry to the list specifically relating to uroscopy, in accordance with his focus on this practice. He also raises the importance of the learned physician by re-ordering the list to make this the first point.

Bibliography

Manuscript Sources

C 241/43/99, National Archives, London.
MS V.b.26 (1), Folger Shakespeare Library, Washington, D.C.
PROB 11/409/101, National Archives, London.
Sloane MS 1954, British Library, London.
Sloane MS 1965, British Library, London.

Printed Works pre-1800

A Briefe Description Of The Notoriovs Life of Iohn Lambe, otherwise called Doctor Lambe. Together with his Ignominious Death. Amsterdam [i.e., London: George Miller?] 1628.

A Rehearsall both straung and true, of hainous and horrible actes committed by Elizabeth Stile, Alias Rockingham, Mother Dutten, Mother Deuell, Mother Margaret, Fower notorious Witches, apprehended at winsore. London: [John Kingston] for Edward White, 1579.

Ars Notoria: The Notory Art Of Solomon. Translated by Robert Turner. London: J. Cottrel to be sold by Martha Harrison, 1657.

Bernard, Richard. *A Gvide To Grand-Ivry Men.* London: Felix Kingston for Edward Blackmore, 1627.

Bonham, Thomas. *The Chyrvrgians Closet.* London: George Miller for Edward Brester, 1630.

Bower, Edmond. *Doctor Lamb Revived.* London: Thomas Wilson[?] for Richard Best and John Place, 1653.

Brian, Thomas. *The Pisse-Prophet, Or, Certaine Pisse-Pot Lectures.* London: E. P. for R. Thrale, 1637.

Casaubon, Meric. *A True & Faithful Relation Of What passed for many Yeers Between Dr. John Dee (A Mathematician of Great Fame in Q. Eliz. and King James their Reignes) and Some Spirits.* London: D. Maxwell for T. Garthwait, 1659.

Cooper, Thomas. *The Mystery Of Witch-craft.* London: Nicholas Okes, 1617.

Cotta, John. *A Short Discoverie Of The Vnobserved Dangers of seuerall sorts of ignorant and vnconsiderate Practisers of Physicke in England.* London: for William Jones and Richard Boyle, 1612.

———. *The Infallible Trve And Assvred Witch.* London: John Legate for Richard Higgenbotham, 1624.

Culpeper, Nicholas. *The English Physician.* London: William Bentley, 1652.

Digby, Kenelm. *A Late Discourse. . . Touching the Cure of Wounds by the Powder of Sympathy.* Translated by R. White. London: R. Lowndes and T. Davies, 1658.

Eusebius. *Ecclesiastical Histories.* London: Thomas Vautroullier, 1577.

F., P. *The Historie of the damnable life, and deserved death of Doctor Iohn Faustus.* London: Thomas Orwin to be sold by Edward White, 1592.

Fludd, Robert. *Anatomiae amphitheatrum.* Frankfurt: Erasmus Kempfer for Theodore de Bry, 1623.

———. *Doctor Flvdds Answer unto M. Foster Or, The Sqvesing Of Parson Fosters Sponge, ordained by him for the wiping away of the Weapon-Salve.* London: for Nathaniel Butter, 1631.

Foreest, Pieter van. *The Arraignment Of Vrines.* Translated by James Hart. London: George Eld for Robert Milbourne, 1623.

Foster, William. *Hoplocrismaspongvs: Or, A Sponge to wipe away the Weapon-Salve.* London: Thomas Cotes for John Grove, 1631.

Gifford, George. *A Discourse of the subtill Practises of Deuilles by Witches and Sorcerers.* London: for Toby Cooke, 1587.

———. *A Dialogve concerning Witches and Witchcraftes.* London: John Windet for Toby Cooke and Mihil Hart, 1593.

Hart, James. *The Anatomie Of Vrines.* London: Richard Field for Robert Milbourne, 1625.

———. *The Diet of The Diseased.* London: John Beale for Robert Allot, 1633.

Henry Cornelius Agrippa his Fourth Book Of Occult Philosophy. Translated by Robert Turner. London: J. C. for John Harrison, 1655.

Heywood, Thomas. *The Hierarchie of the blessed Angells.* London: Adam Islip, 1635.

Holland, Henry. *A Treatise Against VVitchcraft.* Cambridge: John Legate, 1590.

James VI and I. *Daemonologie.* Edinburgh: Robert Waldegrave, 1597.

Jonson, Ben. *The Workes Of Benjamin Ionson.* London: for Richard Meighen, 1641.

Keckermann, Bartholomäus. *Systema Physicvm.* Hanau: William Anthony, 1612.

Mexia, Pedro, Francesco Sansovino, et al. *The Treasvrie Of Avncient And Moderne Times, Containing the Learned Collections, Iudicious Readings, and Memorable Obseruations: Not onely Diuine, Morrall and Phylosophicall. But also Poeticall, Martiall, Politicall, Historicall, Astrologicall, &c.* London: William Jaggard, 1613.

Naudé, Gabriel. *The History of Magick.* Translated by John Davies. London: John Streater, 1657.

Oberndorff, Johann and Francis Herring. *The Anatomyes of the True Physition*. London: for Arthur Johnson, 1602.

Perkins, William. *Fovre Great Lyers*. London: Robert Waldegrave, 1585.

———. *A Discovrse Of The Damned Art of Witchcraft*. Cambridge: Cantrell Legge, 1608.

Potts, Thomas. *The Wonderfvll Discoverie Of Witches In the Covntie of Lancaster*. London: William Stansby for John Barnes, 1613.

Primerose, James. *Popular Errours. Or The Errours of the People In Physick*. Translated by Robert Wittie. London: W. Wilson for Nicholas Bourne, 1651.

Roberts, Alexander. *A Treatise of Witchcraft*. London: Nicholas Okes for Samuel Man, 1616.

Sacchi, Bartolomeo. *The Lives Of The Popes*. Translated by Paul Rycaut. London: for Christopher Wilkinson. 1685.

Scot, Reginald. *The discouerie of witchcraft*. London: [Henry Denham for] William Brome, 1584.

———. *The Discovery of Witchcraft*. London: for Andrew Clark to be sold by Dixy Page, 1665.

Shakespeare, William. *A Midsommer nights dreame*. London: [Richard Bradock] for Thomas Fisher, 1600.

———. *True Chronicle Historie of the life and death of King Lear*. London: [Nicholas Okes] for Nathaniel Butter, 1608.

The Bible. Geneva: Rouland Hall, 1560.

The Brideling, Sadling and Ryding, of a rich Churle in Hampshire, by the subtill practise of one Iudeth Philips, a professed cunning woman, or Fortune teller. London: T. C. to be sold by William Barley, 1595.

The Holy Bible. London: Robert Barker, 1611.

The seuerall Notorious and levvd Cousnages of Iohn West, and Alice West, falsely called the King and Queene of Fayries. London: for Edward Marchant, 1613.

Printed Works post-1800

Ankarloo, Bengkt, Stuart Clark, and William Monter. *Witchcraft and Magic in Europe: The Period of the Witch Trials*. Philadelphia: University of Pennsylvania Press, 2002.

Aubrey, John. *Three Prose Works*. Edited by John Buchanan-Brown. Fontwell: Centaur Press, 1972.

Augustine. *The City of God against the Pagans*. Translated by R. W. Dyson. Cambridge: Cambridge University Press, 1998.

Bailey, Michael D. *Magic and Superstition in Europe: A Concise History from Antiquity to the Present*. Plymouth: Rowman & Littlefield Publishers, 2007.

Batho, G. R. "The Library of the 'Wizard' Earl: Henry Percy Ninth Earl of Northumberland (1564–1632)." *The Library* 15, 4 (1960): 246–61.

Beaufort, D. A. "The Medical Practitioners of Western Sussex in the Early Modern Period: A Preliminary Survey." *Sussex Archaeological Collections* 131 (1993): 139–51.

Beier, Lucinda McCray. *Sufferers and Healers: The Experience of Illness in Seventeenth-Century England.* London: Routledge and Kegan Paul, 1987.

Bellany, Alastair. "The Murder of John Lambe: Crowd Violence, Court Scandal and Popular Politics in Early Seventeenth-Century England." *Past and Present* 200 (2008): 37–76.

Bernard, G. W. and Steven J. Gunn, eds. *Authority and Consent in Tudor England: Essays Presented to C. S. L. Davies.* Aldershot: Ashgate, 2002.

Blécourt, Willem de. "Witch Doctors, Soothsayers and Priests. On Cunning Folk in European Historiography and Tradition." *Social History* 19, 3 (1994): 285–303.

Bodin, Jean. *On the Demon-Mania of Witches.* Translated by Randy A. Scott. Toronto: Centre for Reformation and Renaissance Studies, 2001.

Briggs, Robin. *Witches & Neighbours: The Social and Cultural Context of European Witchcraft.* 2d ed. Oxford: Blackwell, 2002.

Cameron, Euan. *Enchanted Europe: Superstition, Reason, and Religion, 1250–1750.* Oxford: Oxford University Press, 2010.

Carey, John, ed. *Milton: The Complete Shorter Poems.* Harlow: Longman, 2007.

Clark, George. *A History of the Royal College of Physicians of London.* 3 vols. Oxford: Clarendon Press, 1964.

Clark, Stuart. *Thinking With Demons: The Idea of Witchcraft in Early Modern Europe.* Oxford: Oxford University Press, 1997.

Copeland, Clare and Jan Machielsen, eds. *Angels of Light? Sanctity and the Discernment of Spirits in the Early Modern Period.* Leiden: Brill, 2013.

Creager, Angela N. H. and William Chester Jordan, eds. *The Animal/Human Boundary: Historical Perspectives.* Rochester, NY: University of Rochester Press, 2002.

Dandrige, Ross. "Anti-Quack Literature in Early Stuart England." Ph.D. thesis. Queen Mary, University of London, 2012.

Darr, Orna Alyagon. *Marks of an Absolute Witch: Evidentiary Dilemmas in Early Modern England.* Farnham: Ashgate, 2011.

Davies, Owen. *Popular Magic: Cunning-folk in English History.* London: Hambledon Continuum, 2007.

———. *Grimoires: A History of Magic Books.* Oxford: Oxford University Press, 2009.

Davies, Simon, ed. *The Discovery of Witches and Witchcraft: The Writings of the Witchfinders.* Brighton: Puckrel Publishing, 2007.

Debus, Allen G. "Robert Fludd and the Use of Gilbert's *De Magnete* in the Weapon-Salve Controversy." *Journal of the History of Medicine and Allied Sciences* 19, 4 (1964): 389–417.

———. *The Chemical Philosophy: Paracelsian Science and Medicine in the Sixteenth and Seventeenth Centuries.* 2 vols. New York: Science History Publications, 1977.

Dimmock, Matthew, Andrew Hadfield, and Abigail Shinn, eds. *The Ashgate Research Companion to Popular Culture in Early Modern England.* Farnham: Ashgate, 2014.

Dixon, C. Scott, Dagmar Freist, and Mark Greengrass, eds. *Living with Religious Diversity in Early Modern Europe.* Farnham: Ashgate, 2009.

Elmer, Peter. *The Miraculous Conformist: Valentine Greatrakes, the Body Politic and the Politics of Healing in Post Restoration Britain.* Oxford: Oxford University Press, 2012.

Fairfax, Edward. *Daemonologia: A Discourse on Witchcraft.* Edited by William Grainge. London: Frederick Muller, 1971.

Fanger, Claire, ed. *Conjuring Spirits: Texts and Traditions of Medieval Ritual Magic.* University Park: Pennsylvania State University Press, 1998.

Foster, Joseph. *Alumni Oxonienses: The Members of the University of Oxford, 1500–1714.* 4 vols. London: James Parker, 1891.

French, Roger and Andrew Wear, eds. *The Medical Revolution of the Seventeenth Century.* Cambridge: Cambridge University Press, 1989.

Gaskill, Malcolm. "Witchcraft, Politics, and Memory in Seventeenth-Century England." *The Historical Journal* 50.2 (2007): 289–308.

———. "Witchcraft and Evidence in Early Modern England." *Past and Present* 198 (2008): 33–70.

Golden, Richard M., ed. *Encyclopedia of Witchcraft: The Western Tradition.* 4 vols. Santa Barbara: ABC-CLIO, 2006.

Harley, David. "James Hart of Northampton and the Calvinist Critique of Priest-Physicians: An Unpublished Polemic of the Early 1620s." *Medical History* 42 (1998): 362–86.

Jenner, Mark S. R. and Patrick Wallis, eds. *Medicine and the Market in England and Its Colonies, c. 1450–c. 1850.* Basingstoke: Palgrave Macmillan, 2007.

Jones, John Henry, ed. *The English Faust Book.* Cambridge: Cambridge University Press, 1994.

Kassell, Lauren. *Medicine and Magic in Elizabethan London: Simon Forman: Astrologer, Alchemist, & Physician.* Oxford: Oxford University Press, 2005.

Kenyon, G. H. "Petworth Town & Trades 1610–1760." *Sussex Archaeological Collections* 96 (1958): 35–107.

Kieckhefer, Richard. *Magic in the Middle Ages.* Cambridge: Cambridge University Press, 1987.

Klaassen, Frank. *The Transformations of Magic: Illicit Learned Magic in the Later Middle Ages and Renaissance.* University Park: Pennsylvania State University Press, 2013.

Levack, Brian P. *The Witch-Hunt in Early Modern Europe.* 3d ed. Harlow: Pearson Education Ltd., 2006.

———, ed. *The Oxford Handbook of Witchcraft in Early Modern Europe and Colonial America*. Oxford: Oxford University Press, 2013.

Lindemann, Mary. *Medicine and Society in Early Modern Europe*. Cambridge: Cambridge University Press, 2010.

MacDonald, Michael. *Mystical Bedlam: Madness, Anxiety, and Healing in Seventeenth-Century England*. Cambridge: Cambridge University Press, 1981.

MacGregor, Arthur, ed. *Sir Hans Sloane: Collector, Scientist, Antiquary*. London: British Museum Press, 1994.

Marshall, Peter and Alexandra Walsham, eds. *Angels in the Early Modern World*. Cambridge: Cambridge University Press, 2006.

Maxwell-Stuart, P. G. *Wizards: A History*. Stroud: Tempus, 2004.

McLean, Adam, ed. *A Treatise on Angel Magic: Being a Complete Transcription of Ms. Harley 6482 in the British Library*. Grand Rapids: Phanes Press, 1990.

McShane, Angela and Garthine Walker, eds. *The Extraordinary and the Everyday in Early Modern England: Essays in Celebration of the Work of Bernard Capp*. Basingstoke: Palgrave Macmillan, 2010.

Mortimer, Ian. *The Dying and the Doctors: The Medical Revolution in Seventeenth-Century England*. London: Royal Historical Society, 2009.

Pelling, Margaret. *Medical Conflicts in Early Modern London: Patronage, Physicians, and Irregular Practitioners, 1550–1640*. Oxford: Oxford University Press, 2003.

Poole, Robert, ed. *The Lancashire Witches: Histories and Stories*. Manchester: Manchester University Press, 2002.

Raymond, Joad. *Milton's Angels: The Early-Modern Imagination*. Oxford: Oxford University Press, 2010.

———, ed. *Conversations with Angels: Towards a History of Spiritual Communication, 1100–1700*. Basingstoke: Palgrave Macmilllan, 2011.

Roper, Jonathon, ed. *Charms and Charming in Europe*. Basingstoke: Palgrave Macmillan, 2004.

Ryrie, Alec. *The Sorcerer's Tale: Faith and Fraud in Tudor England*. Oxford: Oxford University Press, 2008.

Sangha, Laura. *Angels and Belief in England, 1480–1700*. London: Pickering & Chatto, 2012.

Sharpe, James. *Instruments of Darkness: Witchcraft in England 1550–1750*. London: Penguin, 1997.

Stolberg, Michael. "The Decline of Uroscopy in Early Modern Learned Medicine (1500–1650)." *Early Science and Medicine* 12, 3 (2007): 313–36.

The Key of Solomon the King. Translated and edited by S. Liddell MacGregor Mathers. San Francisco: Weiser Books, 2000.

Thomas, Keith. *Religion and the Decline of Magic*. London: Weidenfeld & Nicolson, 1971.

Vickers, Brian, ed. *Occult & Scientific Mentalities in the Renaissance*. Cambridge: Cambridge University Press, 1984.

Walsham, Alexandra. *Providence in Early Modern England.* Oxford: Oxford University Press, 1999.

Wells, Stanley, ed. *The Oxford Shakespeare: King Lear.* Oxford: Oxford University Press, 2000.

Wilson, Stephen. *The Magical Universe: Everyday Ritual and Magic in Pre-Modern Europe.* London and New York: Hambledon and London, 2000.

Wood, Andy. "'Some banglyng about the customes': Popular Memory and the Experience of Defeat in a Sussex Village, 1549–1640." *Rural History* 25, 1 (2014): 1–14.

Zlatar, A. B. *Reformation Fictions: Polemical Protestant Dialogues in Elizabethan England.* Oxford: Oxford University Press, 2011.

Online sources

The Oxford Dictionary of National Biography. Oxford University Press, available at: www.oxforddnb.com. Cited as *ODNB.*

The Oxford English Dictionary. Oxford University Press, available at: www.oed.com. Cited as *OED.*

INDEX

Notes: Works are listed under their authors. Proper nouns are given in their modern form. Chapters of the Bible are listed under the main entry for the Bible, and are given in their modern form.